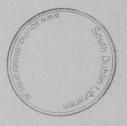

THE
SWEETNESS
OF DOING
NOTHING

Thorsons
An imprint of HarperCollins*Publishers*
1 London Bridge Street
London SE1 9GF
www.harpercollins.co.uk

First published by Thorsons 2020

10 9 8 7 6 5 4 3 2 1

ISBN 9780008366490

Printed and bound at PNB, Latvia

p.4–5 Photo by Dimitry Anikin on Unsplash; p.6 Alaver/Shutterstock.com; p.9 Author's own; p.10 Libero Monterisi/Shutterstock.com; p.17, 18, 21, 22 Author's own; p.27 Simona Sirio/Shutterstock.com; p.28 graphicgeoff/Shutterstock.com; p.30, 31, 33 Author's own; p.35 Chippix/Shutterstock.com; p.37 Author's own; p.40-1; (top left) Daniel Hansen-Pom on Unsplash (top middle) Kate Townsend on Unsplash (right and bottom left) Author's own (bottom middle) Arndale/Shutterstock.com; p.45 Author's own; p.47 Ollirg/Shutterstock.com; p.51, 52, 55, 57, 59 Author's own; p.61 Artens/Shutterstock.com; p.65, 67, 68 Author's own; p.70-1 Shutterstock.com; p.73, 74, 75, 79 Author's own; p.76 Topfoto/EUFD; p.77 Bettmann/Getty Images; p.81, 85, 87 Author's own; p.88 Juan Gomez on Unsplash; p.91, 94 Author's own; p.96-7 Shutterstock.com; p.98 Yulia Grigoryeva/Shutterstock.com; p.101 Author's own; p.102 Roman Kraft on Unsplash; p.103 Ruth Troughton on Unsplash; p.105, 106 Author's own; p.109 Shutterstock.com; p.111, 113 Author's own; p.115 Eric Barbeau on Unsplash; p.116, 119 Author's own; p.121 Vincent Versluis on Unsplash; p.123, 125 Author's own; p.127 Tyler Nix on Unsplash; p.129 (top) Antonio Rossi on Unsplash (bottom) Author's own; p.130 Author's own; p.135 Anna Auza on Unsplash; p.137 Author's own; p.139 La Soon Unsplash; p.140 Alaver/Shutterstock.com; p.142, 145 Stefano Valeri/Shutterstock.com; p.147 Author's own; p.150-1 Villiam.M/Shutterstock.com; p.154-5 Alexandre Rotenberg/Shutterstock.com; p.157, 163 Author's own; p.164 Shyripa Alexandr/Shutterstock.com; p.167, 168, 171, 172, 177, 181, 183, 185, 186 Author's own

SOPHIE MINCHILLI

THE
SWEETNESS
OF DOING
NOTHING

LIVE LIFE THE ITALIAN WAY WITH
DOLCE FAR NIENTE

Thorsons

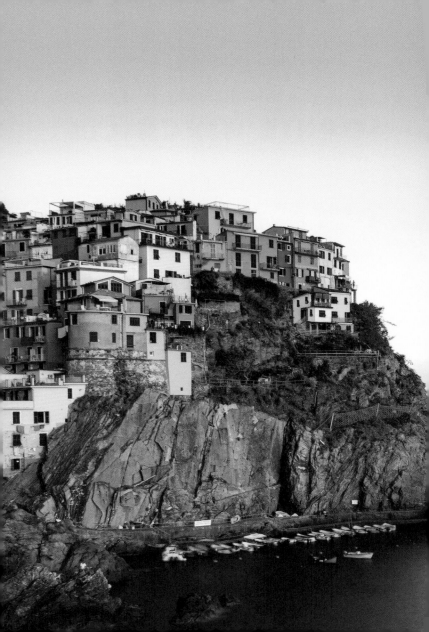

CONTENTS

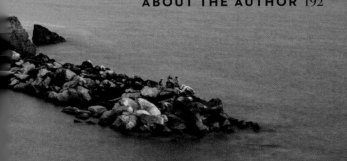

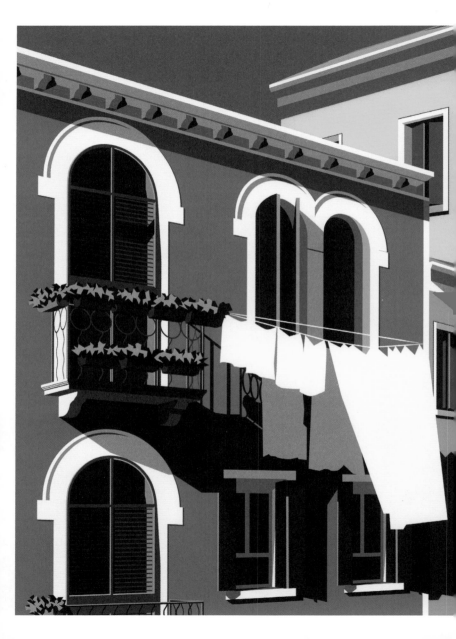

INTRODUCTION

THE ART OF
DOING NOTHING

I WAS BORN AND RAISED IN ITALY, IN THE MIDDLE OF TWO VERY DIFFERENT CULTURES.

My mother is an American, completely in awe of everything Italian. In contrast, my father, a man from the deep Italian south, takes all of the country's beauty and traditions for granted. As for me, growing up in Rome, I took after my father: all the beauty, ancient history and good food that surrounded me were nothing special. As a six-year-old, I didn't think twice about the fact that my classroom in kindergarten overlooked the Colosseum. When the lady in the cafeteria served a different kind of mouthwatering pasta every day for lunch, it was no big deal. And spending endless afternoons running around cobblestoned piazzas, playing hide and seek around the sixteenth-century fountain with my friends after school? Totally normal.

But when school let out for the summer, the city became too hot and – like every other Roman family – we left town to escape the heat. From June to September you'd find me in the countryside in Umbria, where we have a farmhouse, or by the sea in rural Puglia, near my father's family. And it is only now that I realise how much these two places have shaped my personality and the way I live today – just as much as my 'real' life growing up in the city of Rome.

Umbria is a tiny region right in the middle of Italy, known as 'the green heart' because it touches no coastline. Its luscious green hills and winding valleys made it the perfect landscape for me to experience Dolce Far Niente, the sweet art of doing nothing, at a very young age. Summer holidays – which were a full three months – were spent at our restored farmhouse on the outskirts of a tiny village. My most vivid memories are of mornings spent at

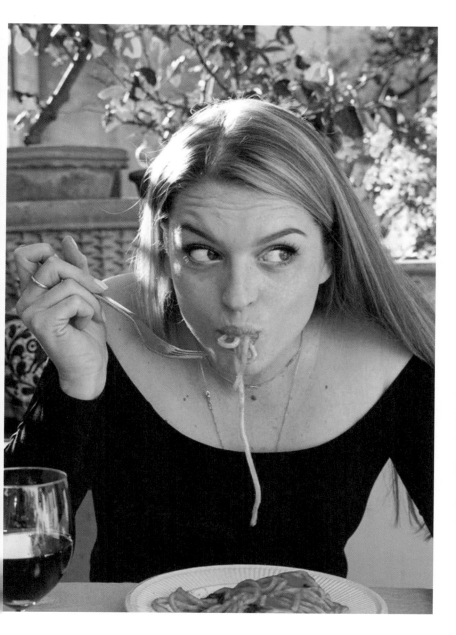

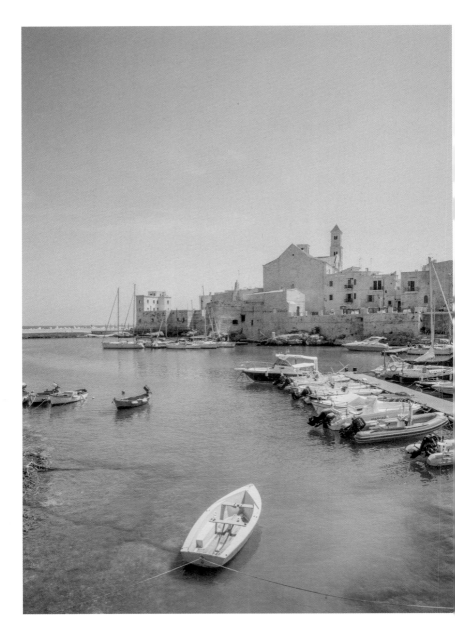

our neighbours' home, just down the dirt road. My mother would drop me off there, along with my sister, Emma, every day right before breakfast. Being a writer, my mother worked from home, so her writing time came while we were out. My father, an architect, would commute back and forth to his office in Rome.

Emma and I couldn't wait to be dropped off every morning at our neighbours' very much working farm, filled with an extended family and animals. Once we were there, Daniela, our babysitter, would join in our very special routine which has stuck with me ever since: a long, slow breakfast with Sandra (Daniela's mum) on the front porch. Then it was time for 'chores'. The first stop was going to the chicken coop to pick eggs with Settimio (Daniela's father), then taking a walk to her Uncle Angelo's to say hi to the cows and sheep before walking to the stream-fed fountain to visit her aunt, Lina, while she washed the family's laundry by hand. The highlight of the day (and you'll see this will be a recurring theme in this book) was heading back to Sandra's kitchen where we'd pick out a pasta shape for lunch. While Sandra made us lunch, Settimio would take us to sit on the *ceppa*, a homemade stoop under a big, shady tree. Finally, Sandra would shout *'a tavola'* out the window, and we all gathered for lunch, my sister and I smiling and chatting about our long morning and all the people and animals we had seen.

The pace of the days was always slow (very slow), and what our summers there taught us was that you should never be rushed. The best things in life need to be enjoyed slowly, and with a smile.

Like all Italian families, we also spent some time at the sea. During the final weeks of the summer holidays, when my father closed up his office, we packed our bags and made the long journey south to the region of Puglia, which is the heel of the 'boot' that is Italy. My father was born and raised there, and it's known for some of the most gorgeous beaches, small white towns, luscious cheeses and the freshest, tastiest vegetables in the whole country. My family would meet up with my paternal grandparents at the very tip of the region to spend a full ten days at the beach – eating, napping and playing the last summer days away.

If I failed to appreciate all this as a child, as I grew older, I realised just how lucky I was. The more time I spent away from Italy (summers studying abroad throughout high school, followed by university in England), the more I understood that looking at the Colosseum during breaktimes at school, picking eggs with a family of farmers in the middle of Umbria and eating freshly picked watermelon on one of the most beautiful beaches in Italy were really quite extraordinary.

After high school, I made the decision to move to London to get a university degree. While I loved the novelty and rush of the big city, along with all the wonderful opportunities London was giving me, I also missed Italy with all my heart: the endless Sunday lunches with my family, meeting my childhood friends for a drink before dinner, walking around my neighbourhood and seeing familiar faces on every corner, drinking coffee each morning at the place I had been going to since I was a baby and the absolutely gorgeous architecture and art at every turn. I understood, for the first time, that I had grown up in an open-air museum filled with beauty. So I finished my degree, packed my bags and said goodbye to London. I was going back to R(h)ome.

After a couple years back in Rome, I finally managed to turn my love for Italy into a full-time job: together with my mother, Elizabeth Minchilli, I lead food tours around my favourite neighbourhoods in Rome, the places where I grew up, running around as a child. I wanted to share all the things I previously took for granted with people from all over the world. And funnily enough, most of the things I love about Rome have to do with food: old-fashioned bakeries, cookie shops, open-air markets, local men sitting outside coffee bars playing cards. But it's never *just* the food I am sharing. It's everything that surrounds every bite we take: the culture and way of life.

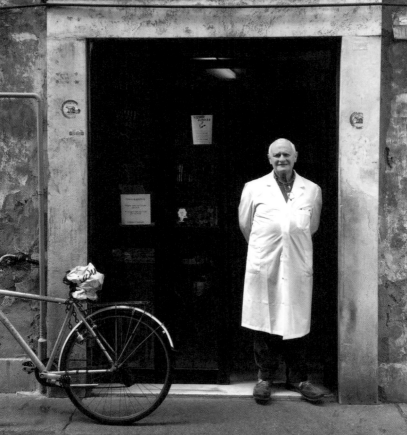

But while this Italian way of life is attractive to many people who dream about architectural beauty, seemingly endless meals, music and gorgeous little towns, it is also sometimes criticised. I often hear people say that Italians are lazy, that they don't like to work. And terms like *la dolce vita*, *sprezzatura*, *la grande bellezza* and Dolce Far Niente feature in countless movies, books and conversations.

In today's world, most of us have made too much space for things we don't actually need, constantly inviting clutter into our physical and psychological space. Keeping busy often makes us feel important and purposeful. If we are not occupied all the time, we tend to feel useless or lazy. To be considered successful, we must produce something. Status is reflected in the amount of running around we do, the number of items checked off our to-do lists.

But Italians have a different approach. Most understand that keeping constantly busy often leads to anxiety, stress-related diseases and burnout. Dolce Far Niente – 'the sweet art of doing nothing' – is a state of complete idleness or blissful relaxation. Italians have figured out a way of being in the moment with such joy and blissfulness that they are not 'looking forward' to anything else. And while they may seem lazy from the outside, what I hope to convey with this book is that when they are apparently 'doing nothing', they are actually doing a lot.

Over the years, I've slowly learned that when Italians take a full lunch break with friends in the middle of the week, long *aperitivi* at the end of the day or spend their Sundays just lounging in the sun, they are not 'doing nothing'. They have learned that fallow time is necessary to grow and produce – anything from children to a successful business. To work better, we need to rest, laugh, read and reconnect. We should not feel embarrassed when 'doing nothing', but think of it as an important tool that helps us to enjoy the best life we can possibly have.

Yet it is precisely this art of 'doing nothing' that so frequently comes under fire from both Italians themselves and people abroad.

This misconception became most apparent to me through a negative response to some of the pictures on my Instagram page. (I should mention that Instagram has become a wonderful tool for me to show the world the Italy that I love and grew up with – everything from my neighbourhood, my favourite vendor at the market and the postman I have known all my life, to the barista who has been making me coffee every morning for the past twenty-nine years, all of whom I consider national treasures.) At first glance, my pictures might all seem very similar: men or women from all over Italy just sitting around, apparently doing nothing. But on closer inspection, you will see that every one of them has a story (I write a caption and story below each photograph), and that man who is seemingly doing nothing is actually taking a break after years and years of back-breaking work. Still, some people feel I am showing an Italy that isn't real, an Italy made of older lazy people who don't work. To them, I should be showing a younger Italy, the one that puts on a suit and tie every morning and commutes to an office.

While at first I felt hurt, I almost immediately realised that none of the people I've photographed have been staged or set up, and so they are very much part of the 'real' Italy. This is *exactly* the Italy I grew up with, the one I love and the one I show my clients on my food tours. I also realised that while Italy is, of course, a modern country with offices and people in suits and ties, it also manages to keep old traditions alive – all thanks to these older people I photograph. These men and women, living in their small towns, doing what they have done for years, make up my Italy.

The art of 'Dolce Far Niente' has been around since the Roman Empire, and even though Italy is very different from north to south, this is the one aspect of life that brings everyone together, no matter their age or the region they grew up in.

WHAT DOLCE FAR NIENTE MEANS TO ME

SINCE THE CONCEPT OF DOLCE FAR NIENTE IS SO BROAD AND SO ALL-ENCOMPASSING, IT WAS DIFFICULT AT FIRST TO KNOW HOW TO CONVEY IT IN AN ORGANISED WAY. BUT I FINALLY SAW THAT THE ART OF DOING NOTHING COULD BEST BE EXPLAINED BY LOOKING AT WHAT ARE, FOR ME, THE THREE MOST IMPORTANT ASPECTS OF ITALIAN LIFE: FOOD; FAMILY AND FRIENDS; AND LEISURE.

So, after a brief dip into Italy's past and its geography, we will explore food – probably the cornerstone of Italian life: Sunday lunches, shopping at the market, eating with the seasons, pasta, pizza, wine and cheese. Since food is so central to Italian culture, and I am typically Italian when it comes to food, it's no wonder that this is also the longest chapter in the book. And hardly surprising too, given that – in true 'Dolce Far Niente' style – I've managed to successfully transform my love for food into my work. In this chapter, I will explain what it's like to cook and eat in Italy, and also give you tips and recipes on how to bring some of that delicious magic into your own home.

Next come family and friends. The time that Italians spend with both family and friends – which, to an outsider, can seem like 'doing nothing' – forms the foundation of their sense of contentment. All Italians have a deep understanding about the value of tight family bonds, how friendships will often last a lifetime and the importance of growing old surrounded by love. Tied in with this is the role of women in Italy and, most significantly, the

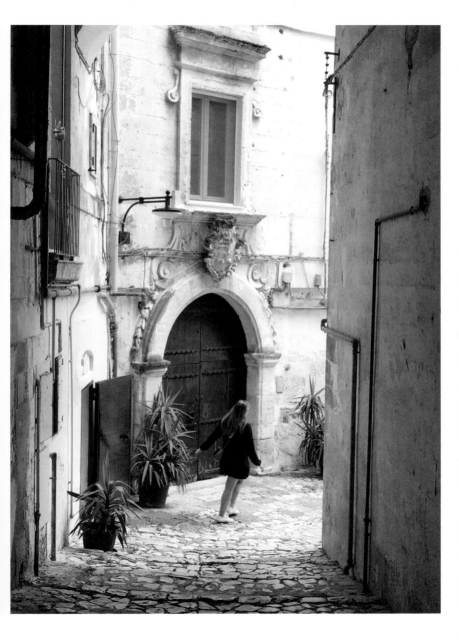

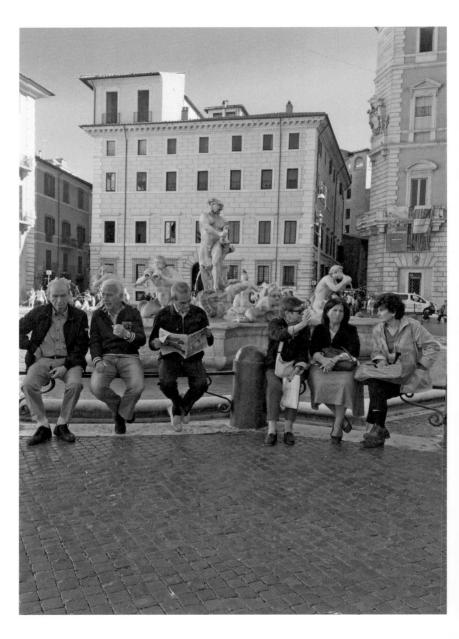

god-like figure known as *la mamma*. Through understanding why family and friends are so central to an Italian's everyday life, I hope that you will be inspired to create and maintain stronger bonds with your own loved ones.

Italians take their downtime very seriously. So in the final chapter, 'Leisure', I explore how Italians have perfected the art of relaxing when not working (and often *while* working); activities like going to the beach, taking long walks, meeting for a coffee or drink, listening to music and playing endless card games are not just add-ons, but essential aspects of daily life. After a lifetime in Italy, I have come to know countless ways in which Italians like to relax, drawing a clear line between work and fun, while at the same time combining them, so both become enjoyable. As well as describing such 'activities', I will also give you a few tips on how you can adopt some of them and blend them into your own daily life.

LEARNING TO SLOW DOWN

There are so many aspects of Italian culture that I think are key to living a happier and more fulfilled life. First of all, we need to remember that life is indeed very short. But rather than meaning that we should rush through it to accomplish as many things as possible, we should take it slowly, appreciating each day as if it were the last. Whether it's spending an extra hour at the dinner table chatting with our loved ones or a whole afternoon playing a 'useless' card game with our friends, these are the ordinary moments that will bring us happiness in the long run and remain ingrained in our memories for ever.

We've been conditioned to believe that we need to achieve 'perfection' by having a successful career, making lots of money and having the perfect body and clothes. Sure, these are all things that may bring us immediate happiness, but not for the long haul. Technology and social media also play a big part in feeding our anxiety about achieving perfection. We are constantly bombarded with images of people travelling to luxurious and exotic destinations, wearing state-of-the-art designer shoes while eating the latest food trend on the rooftop of the coolest bar in town. However, we often forget that this is not reality: social media and real life are two very different things. What people don't usually show on their social-media platforms is what goes on behind the scenes – when they are spending their afternoon in their pyjamas, reading a book or sipping on a coffee with a friend they haven't seen in five years, chatting about life. I'm not saying that the rise in technology and social media is a bad thing (I love it and have a job thanks to it) – just that it has come into our lives way too fast, and we need to learn how to separate it from real life in order to let our minds live more peacefully.

We need to accept the fact that not everyone is perfect and that there are days when we are allowed to feel sad, days we don't feel like going to work and days when we feel like eating more than we are 'supposed' to. We also need to remember that feelings of anxiousness and overwhelm are perfectly normal, and we are the only ones who can make it better for ourselves.

What I want to try to convey with this book is that we all need to slow down, take our time and enjoy the simpler things in life. We need to retrain ourselves to be bored again. Think about what your grandparents would do when they weren't working. Nothing much, probably. But that 'nothingness' made them happy and definitely didn't leave them feeling like they were missing out on something else. They were simply there, enjoying the peace of the moment.

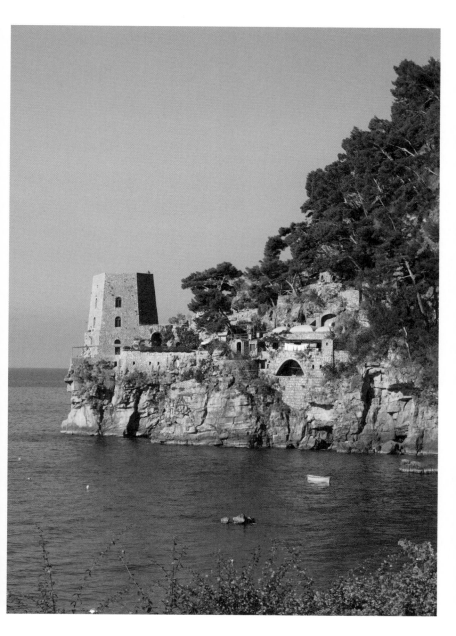

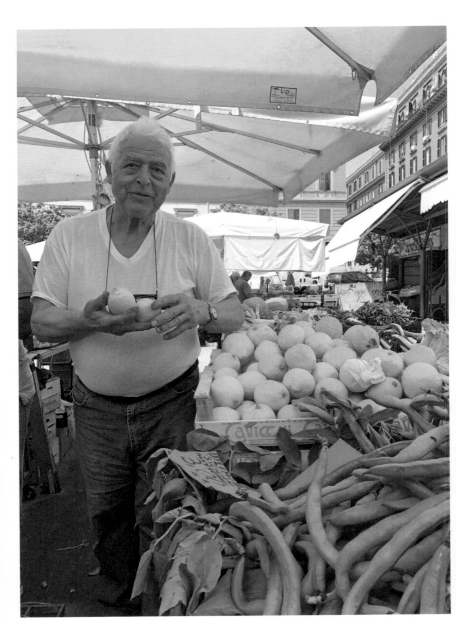

This book is my love letter to Italy. The information in these pages is a mixture of memories and stories I've acquired from friends, family and casual encounters. I didn't want to produce yet another travel guide to add to the thousands already out there. Some of the Italian habits, 'rules' and customs I describe are funny, some less so, but they all reflect what I love most about Italy. In other words: it's personal.

My hope is that you will finish the book with a deeper knowledge of what it is to grow up and live like an Italian, and a good idea of what you can do to bring some of the 'sweet art of doing nothing' to your own life. You will learn that there is no real separation between work and leisure – the two should come together and blend peacefully – and your day-to-day actions should be influenced by your instincts and not by routines and obligations.

I also hope that after reading this book you will be smitten by my country and all the little things that keep me falling in love with it more and more every day. I feel so lucky to have grown up in such a beautiful (and sometimes messy) culture.

A life in Italy can teach you many lessons, but the most important one is to enjoy every single moment, and live life to the fullest, no matter what. Never forget what is important to you and smile your life away.

HOW IT ALL BEGAN:
A LITTLE BACKGROUND HISTORY

When thinking about Italy, you probably envisage beautiful scenery, delicious food, music, art, Vespas and mouthwatering wine. Few other nations have produced as many great painters, sculptors, composers, writers, movie directors and architects, and our small peninsula boasts more UNESCO cultural treasures than any other. Italy's inhabitants created the first libraries, banks, medical schools and universities. Perhaps, coming from a past of violence, oppression and natural disasters, Italians figured out that the best way to counteract the negativity was through architectural beauty, delicious food, good music and joy.

While I certainly don't want to bore you with a lengthy history lesson, I do need to mention a few important facts, just to put things in perspective, because Italy's rich history deeply impacts the way we live today.

The art of Dolce Far Niente is nothing new: the concept of appreciating the moment has been around since the Roman Empire. Granted, most people didn't have much leisure time on their hands back then (they were busy creating an empire and trying not to starve, after all), but they still had a couple of hours a day to relax in the baths and a few days a month for entertaining spectacles such as circuses, gladiator fights and theatre shows. The Romans even had a word for this in Latin – *otium* – referring to leisure time in which a person can enjoy eating, playing, resting, contemplation and the pursuit of academic endeavours.

Roman baths are a perfect example of Dolce Far Niente. Public baths were a common feature in most Roman cities – often huge and including a variety of rooms, each offering different temperatures and spaces for socialising while not doing much else. These baths were a sort of escape from life's everyday struggles and some of the most important ruins in Rome today are, in fact, the ancient baths of Caracalla.

Another example of the Roman concept of *otium* are the villas that wealthy Romans built on the outskirts of cities. As the Roman Empire expanded, many Romans became rich in a very short time. One of the first things they did was to construct hugely extravagant country villas. Previously, most people had lived in the towns or cities, leaving the countryside to the farmers and slaves. Now, suddenly, people realised that properties surrounded by nature – featuring decorative fountains, flowers and herbs, intricate mosaics and frescoes – could be the perfect setting for relaxing and entertaining friends. The Romans understood that to be able to work better, they needed to shut off their brains for a while. That in order to create beauty, they needed to establish the correct balance of work and play. Important figures like Pliny and Cicero praised leisure time and encouraged a life of contemplation and meditation.

Even though the Roman Empire ended up crumbling, its influence became deeply embedded in the Italian DNA. People in Italy (and all over the world) still do as the Romans did: indulging in good food and soothing music, cheering on their team at games, taking their time over meals, sipping on delicious wine while laughing with friends and family, respecting their elders and enjoying walks in nature.

Between the fall of the Roman Empire and unification in the nineteenth century, Italy was split into realms, duchies, municipalities, often at war with each other. If you've been to Italy, you may have noticed how very different people are in Venice compared to those in Rome or Naples, or the people in Sicily compared to those in Milan. These differences are due, partly, to the late unification of the country, but mostly to the country's natural geographical divisions. Being a peninsula, Italy is surrounded by three different seas, has borders with several countries, including France and Switzerland in the north, a backbone of mountains running through the middle, endless lakes and rivers and numerous islands. If you asked me which my favourite part of Italy is, I probably could not give you an answer.

I have been living here for twenty-nine years and discover something new (and beautiful) every time I get in the car and drive.

Each region has specific dialects, recipes and traditions. But even though the country is still very much divided between north, central and south, the one thing that brings Italians together is a zest for life. They put so much enthusiasm into all they do that at the end of the day they need to feel a state of complete and utter mindfulness. No matter their background or economic status, every Italian will tell you they have a passion, whether that's salsa lessons on the weekends, fishing with friends, enjoying the summer breeze on a stoop.

Dolce Far Niente means different things to different people, but it's definitely possible to bring it into your life one way or another; from a cookery lesson on the weekend to reading a book on the couch – you just need to find your way. Life is precious and Italians take every opportunity to live theirs to the fullest. They work hard at minimising what's considered boring or mundane, while maximising whatever is delightful. Their skill for brushing off the hardships of life and making them somehow seem 'lighter' is one I've always admired deeply.

❋ ❋ ❋ ❋ ❋

The subjects I write about here are all based on my personal experiences, travels and encounters and may not be representative of all Italians. To get to know all of Italy would take an entire lifetime, and even though I was born and raised here, I am still learning about it every day; but the art of Dolce Far Niente seems to be a part of every Italian to some extent, and so this book is the perfect way to introduce you to Italian living.

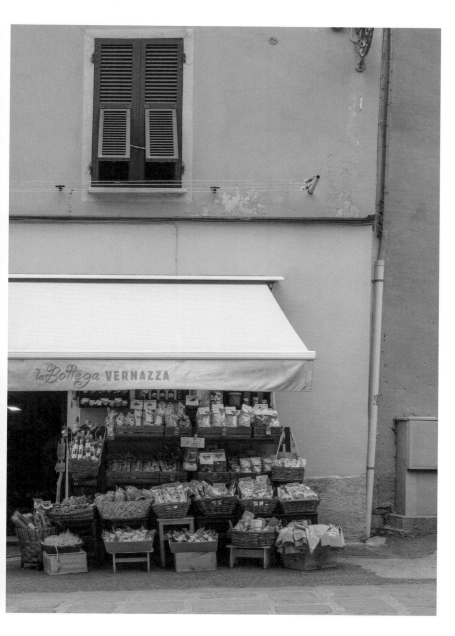

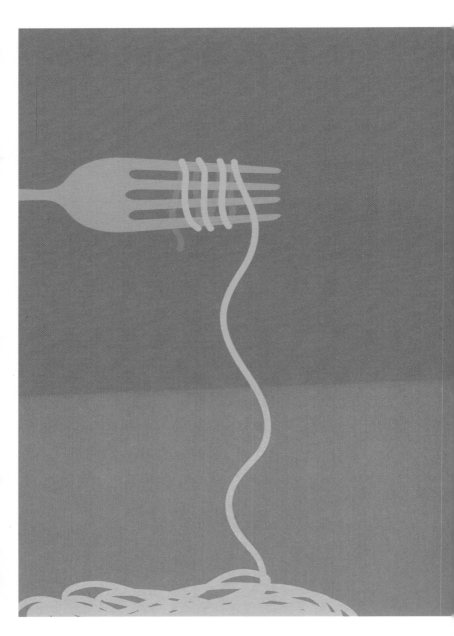

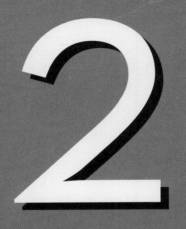

FOOD

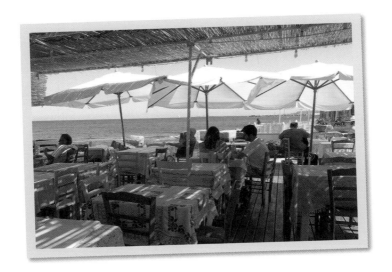

FOOD

Il cibo

Even if you've never been to Italy, you've probably eaten – and enjoyed – Italian food, and I'm sure that words like pasta, pizza, tiramisu and mozzarella sound familiar to most readers.

Italian cuisine is one of the most popular in the world. It is known worldwide and has inspired countless chefs and cookery writers abroad. While at first it may seem that food has nothing to do with Dolce Far Niente, you will see, after reading this chapter, that it is a fundamental part of it.

We all know we like Italian food because it tastes good, but you might be surprised to find out that it's one of the most important aspects of daily life here in Italy. I'm not exaggerating when I say it's all people speak, think and worry about, almost all day long (kind of like the weather for the Brits). What will you be eating for dinner? Whose mother makes the best tomato

30

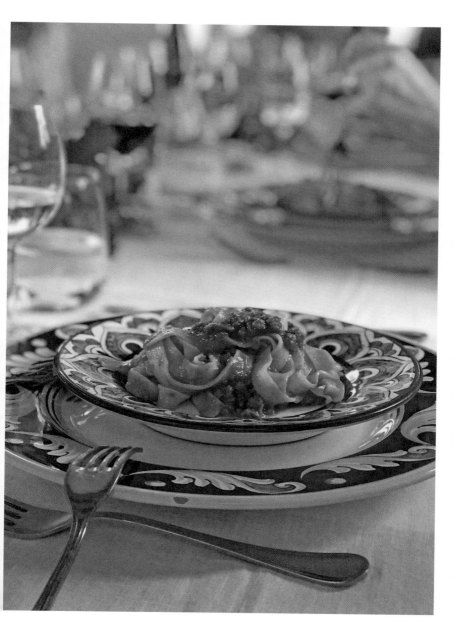

sauce? Do you use pancetta or *guanciale*? Pecorino or parmigiano? The conversations are endless and the ensuing fights extremely common.

One of the reasons why people in Italy are so obsessed with food is because it's so strongly associated with family. Recipes are passed down through generations and become a real part of a family's identity and tradition. Italians don't see food as just sustenance – it's culture, emotion, beauty, family and, quite frankly, an embellishment to daily life. Most Italians can't imagine a life without delicious food, and normal day-to-day tasks are often 'decorated' either with the addition of food or conversations about food to come. Food in Italy is never just fuel to keep you going; it's not meant to end hunger – it's meant to satisfy it, slowly.

And of course, something this important – and pleasurable – is intimately tied to the concept of Dolce Far Niente. A meal is always something to be savoured. Even if it is a lunch break at work, Italians sit down and are expected to enjoy the food and wine that is in front of them. And, wherever possible, with a little companionship and good conversation on the side.

TAKING TIME OUT FOR FOOD

While studying in London for my degree in communications, I had a few jobs, including an office position. On my first day there, I noticed everyone was eating their lunch at their computers, even though there was a big communal table in the next room. Confused, I ate alone on my first day there, but decided the next day that I would ask one of the others in the office to join me at that big table. In time, others followed, and we made it our little 'Italian' tradition to eat lunch together every day.

Many people think there isn't enough time in the day for a slow-paced lunch break sitting down at a table, but if you actually think about it, if you leave your desk for 30 minutes, will the world come to an end? By enjoying your lunch slowly and having a conversation with a co-worker you will give your brain a rest and work better afterwards. Think of it as an investment! Shutting your brain off at meals and focusing only on the food that is in front of you (and on the person you're with, if you're eating in company) is integral to Dolce Far Niente. A meal should be treated as a sacred and somewhat healing moment in your busy day.

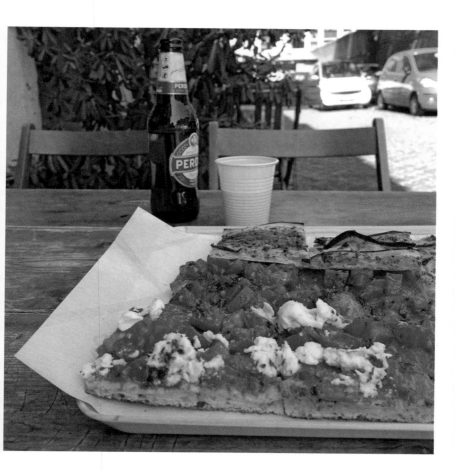

WHAT ARE THE KIDS EATING?
Cosa mangiano i bambini?

Italians are also obsessed with kids. They just love them. Parents bring them along to any occasion and random people will stop and admire your baby in the street, giving you a nice '*quanto è bello*!' ('he's so cute'). Italians expect kids to be involved in mealtime experiences, whether they're long, fancy or casual – and I love them for it.

Italians learn to eat and enjoy the food that is in front of them at a very young age. When out for dinner in any Italian city, you might notice there are children everywhere, no matter the time of day or night or the type of restaurant. Most will have a few high chairs available, but none will have a children's menu. I'd never even seen one before I travelled to the United States for the first time.

Whether at home or at a restaurant, Italian children always sit at the dinner table with grown-ups. There is no 'kids' table'. This means they grow up sitting on the laps of grandparents, parents and uncles. They learn to sit, eat 'grown-up' food, talk and listen simultaneously and to speak loud enough so that everyone else at the table can hear them.

Some of my own first (and best) memories are food-related, and even though I have a terrible memory, I can still remember my first bites of pasta, prosciutto, parmigiano and lettuce. (Who knew my first taste of salad would be ingrained in my memory for ever?)

Outside of my home, a few of my earliest food recollections are from restaurants, but mostly it is our school lunches that I remember. I went to a public elementary school in Rome where we ate two meals a day: a mid-morning snack and lunch. Lunch was a long affair (or at least it seemed so to me, as a small child) with three courses. We were all made to sit together at a long table and couldn't leave until we'd eaten all our food. The *primo* (first course) was usually a soup or pasta, while the *secondo* was meat or fish,

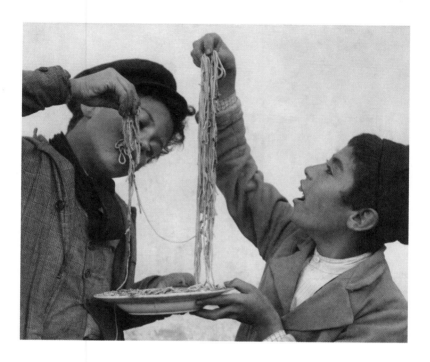

accompanied by some vegetables. Every meal would end with a piece of fruit, and on one special day a week we would get *gelato*. As a kid, I dreaded having to eat things like lentils, aubergine, artichokes and spinach, even though portions were small. Today, as a grown woman, I understand the importance of those long lunches filled with seasonal vegetables: they were teaching us how to act and eat like grown-ups – a skill I am so very grateful for today. They also taught me another important life lesson: meals are meant to be enjoyed at the table, surrounded by friends or family.

SNACK TIME
Merenda

I'm afraid there is no direct translation into English for the word *merenda*, but the closest thing would be a snack. *Fare la merenda* (to have a snack) is an important part of any Italian kid's day. It usually happens mid-afternoon, and as you grow up, it becomes sort of shameful to admit you still have *merenda* (not for me, though – I can't live without it). It usually consists of something sweet, accompanied by a cup of coffee for grown-ups and a juice for kids. To me, having *merenda* every day is an essential part of the Dolce Far Niente way of living: taking a break mid-afternoon to have a comforting snack that reminds you of your childhood? I can't think of anything more soothing. Some of the most popular *merende* in Italy are:

- **Pane e Nutella** – a slice of bread smothered in the famous chocolate-hazelnut spread. I would only be allowed to have this on very special occasions, and I can clearly remember sneaking into the kitchen with my best friend (we were eight years old) and eating it by the spoonful, directly from the jar. We got in big trouble.
- **A slice of homemade cake** – the most popular is *ciambellone* or *crostata*. The first is a very simple ring cake, while the second is jam tart. Every respectable home in Italy has one of these cakes on their kitchen counter.
- **Gelato** – usually only in the summer months, but can be acceptable in the winter as well, since we often have warm, sunny days.
- **Panino** – some kids prefer savoury over sweet; a panino is literally just a sandwich, that can be stuffed with whatever you feel like: cheese, meat, tomatoes or tuna.

Back in the day, it was more common for both kids and adults to partake in the *merenda* ritual, especially if you lived on a farm and had long days

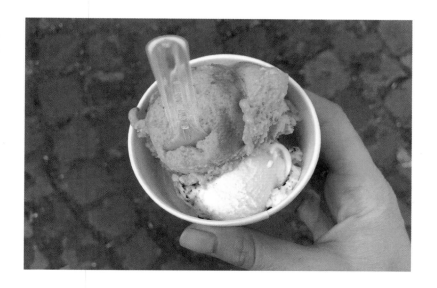

out in the fields. In general, people used to eat less food, so it was normal to get hungry mid-afternoon. I always like to hear what people from older generations liked to have for *merenda*.

When my mom was out of town, my dad would feed me and my sister what he grew up eating for *merenda* as a kid: *pane, burro e alici* for me, (toasted bread, butter and anchovies; yes, I was the weird child who ate anchovies) and *pane e olio* (toasted bread and olive oil) for my sister. To this day, I still think a piece of toasted bread with some butter and an anchovy is the best invention ever for snack time.

One of the major differences between the Italian *merenda* and just snacking, is that it is a fixed event in the day. It doesn't simply happen when you are hungry, grabbing whatever is nearest. Stopping for *merenda* happens as far away from normal mealtime as possible (so as not to interfere with your appetite for a real meal) and is usually a shared, social occasion. A chance to stop what you are doing (work, play, school) and take a break.

LUNCH BREAK
Pausa pranzo

In Italy, the idea of a workday coming to a complete and abrupt stop for a food break is completely normal.

Lunch is the most important and biggest meal in any Italian's day. It's a chance to shut their brains off from work, have a chat with family or friends and enjoy a proper meal sitting down at a table. In the past, most people used to leave their place of work to go home for lunch. Today, things have changed (especially in the big cities), and most people will take their lunch break at a bar or restaurant, not at home.

For kids, up until about the age of ten or eleven, lunch is served at school, but I vividly remember after that, getting out of school every day at 2 pm and making my way home to meet my parents and sister for lunch. My dad would come back from the office and my mom would stop whatever she was doing and make the whole family a beautiful and delicious meal. For most people in Italy, lunch is the opportunity to have a big plate of pasta, while dinner will be something lighter, like a soup or some fish or meat accompanied by a side of greens.

Going back a couple of generations, my grandmother always tells me stories about the days when she would spend the whole morning cooking for my grandfather, so that he would have a warm meal waiting for him when he returned from the office. After eating and taking a nap, he would then go back to work.

Some of my childhood memories include very-early-morning phone calls from my grandma, wanting to speak to my mother to discuss (and share ideas) on what she could make for lunch that day. After the phone call, my *nonna* would make her way to the market to shop for lunch, and later start cooking.

Today, things are very different and, especially in bigger cities, most women no longer spend their entire morning preparing lunch at home. People have started to eat out at the 'bar'.

THE BAR
Il bar

After a short five-minute walk around Rome, you will notice that every single corner of the city has two things: a church and a bar. However, a bar in Italy is not only a place that serves alcohol, but a sort of magical 'home away from home' (as a friend once put it: 'A bar is like a home without a key'), where people can satisfy their needs, from breakfast in the morning to lunch and after-work drinks in the evening.

At lunchtime, most bars will serve a variety of foods, including a few pastas, a soup and some vegetables. Sandwiches come in the form of cute little triangles, called *tramezzini*, comprising fluffy white bread filled with tuna and artichokes, mozzarella and tomato, boiled egg and salami and much more.

Once you pick your bar in Italy (this usually happens at a very young age), you stick with it for ever. The owners know you like your parents do, and when you sit down for lunch or coffee, you don't even have to ask for anything – they already know what you want. You trust them with your lunch as you would trust the food that comes out of your grandma's kitchen.

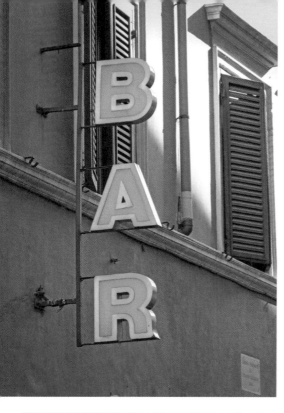
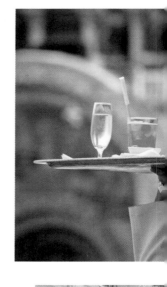
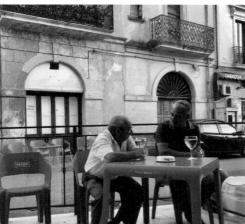
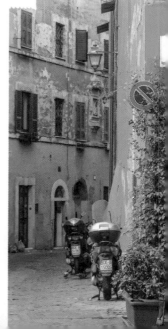

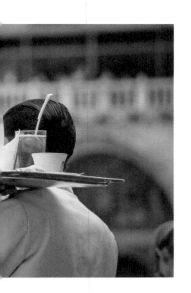

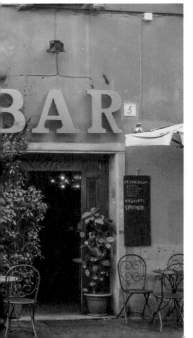

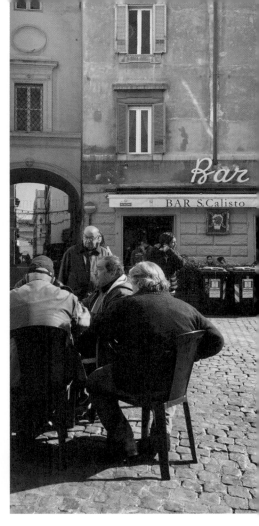

SUNDAY LUNCH
Pranzo della Domenica

The most sacred of all meals in Italy is Sunday lunch. Sunday is the day when all family members and groups of friends come together for a long (and I mean *really* long) meal. Every Sunday, between 12.30 and 1 pm, piazzas and streets will empty out, churches will close their doors after mass and bars will serve their last drinks before people make their way home or to a restaurant for the holy meal that is Sunday lunch.

This is the kind of meal where people indulge in four courses. In a restaurant it would be something like this:

- *Antipasto* – Italian for starter. Usually, you can ask the waiter to bring '*antipasti misti per il tavolo*', which translates to 'a mixture of starters for the whole table'. Depending on where you are in Italy, this might include cheeses, cured meats, seafood, *crostini* or *bruschette*, cured vegetables and fried everything.
- *Primo* – this means first, and in Italy the first and most important thing is always pasta. If you are in northern Italy, you will be able to find fresh homemade pasta, risotto or polenta. In Rome, you will find my favourites: *carbonara*, *amatriciana* (see pages 48 and 49) and *gricia*, all made with *pastasciutta* (dried pasta). In southern Italy, you will find a mixture of fresh and dried pasta, some of the most famous being orecchiette from the region of Puglia. During the winter months, soup is also very common.
- *Secondo* – meaning second, a *secondo* is usually a meat or fish course. Remember that these are never accompanied by a side in Italy. You have to ask for it. The *contorni* (side dishes) vary from season to season, so make sure you ask the waiter what they have that day – you might be in for a delicious and seasonal surprise. And remember: salad is never a starter.

- *Dolce* – a perfect Sunday lunch always ends with something sweet, and depending on where you are in Italy (and the season), you will be able to find all kinds of desserts. Remember to also ask for an *amaro* after your dessert – a bitter alcoholic drink made of wild herbs; Italians believe that slowly sipping a glass (or two) helps you digest your food.

If you are cooking a Sunday lunch at home, chances are somebody (most likely the grandma or mum of the family), will be preparing a tomato and meat sauce for the pasta, known as *sugo*. During the week, most people will make a quick vegetarian sauce, but on Sundays they indulge, adding meat, meaning it will also take longer to cook. Traditionally, women will wake up very early to start the cooking. I can assure you that if you take a walk anywhere in Italy on a Sunday morning, the aroma of the *sugo* is the first thing you will smell.

If you are invited to a Sunday lunch at someone's house, always remember to show up with a tray of pastries or cookies. Actual traffic jams form on a Sunday in Italy in the couple of hours before lunch because of all the people frantically making their way to pastry shops.

SUNDAY TOMATO SAUCE
Sugo della Domenica

Each family has their own recipe, which has been passed down from generation to generation. Here is one I learned from my *nonna* in southern Italy, the smell of which immediately takes me back to Sunday mornings in Puglia.

When the *sugo* is ready, let it sit for an hour or more (the longer it sits the better). To serve, you can either place the meat on top of each plate of pasta, or eat it after the pasta as a *secondo*. I usually prefer to eat the pasta only with the sauce and then eat the meat later, but everyone likes it differently in my family, so every Sunday lunch was always punctuated by a discussion on who did it the 'right' way.

The trick to making this sauce delicious is in getting really good ingredients: make sure you have the best tomato passata you can possibly find, as well as high-quality olive oil and meat.

SERVES 4

4 thin slices veal
50g grated pecorino (or parmigiano)
1 garlic clove, finely chopped
a few parsley and basil leaves
olive oil (enough for a full layer on the base, at least 5–6 tbsp)
4 fresh sausages
125ml red wine
1 bottle tomato passata (about 750g)

1. Prepare the *involtini*: little veal rolls which will be cooked in the sauce. Lay out the veal slices on a counter and pound them to thin them down.
2. Place some of the cheese, garlic and herbs in the centre of each slice. Roll up and secure with a toothpick
3. Pour some olive oil in the bottom of a pan. Once it has heated add the *involtini* and the sausages and let them brown.
4. Once the meat has browned, add the red wine and let it evaporate, then pour in the tomato passata and cook for 2–3 hours. If the sauce seems to dry out at any point, you can add some water.

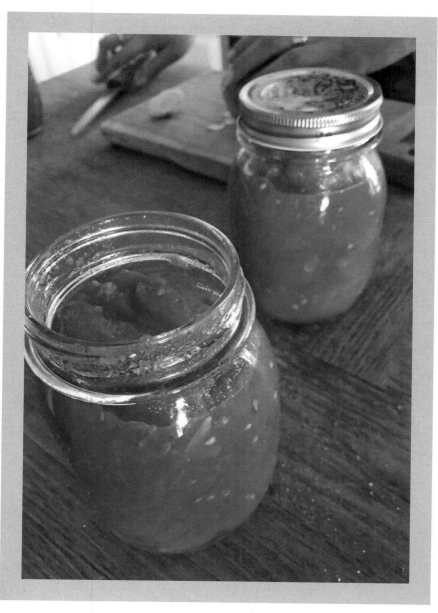

THE COOKING OF THE PEOPLE
Cucina popolare

If you ask anyone in Italy where the best food can be found, they will answer *'a casa, con Nonna'*: 'at home, with Grandma'. And if you insist on asking where else one could find that level of deliciousness, they will tell you the restaurant right next to their building serves the second-best food to Grandma's.

Italians find comfort in tradition and would choose their *nonna*'s meatballs in tomato sauce any day over the newer restaurants that have popped up all over the place. The fact that so many extended families still manage to live together under one roof means that *nonne* are still cooking, and the rest of the family has learned to eat and cook thanks to them. This is why *cucina popolare* (or *cucina povera*) – the cooking style of what used to be the 'lower class' of society – has managed not only to survive, but thrive. Whatever you had in your pantry and whatever was cheapest at the market was what you used to cook a meal for your family. The most humble and delicious dishes in Italy are those made with simple local ingredients, hence so many regional recipes have stood the test of time.

The cooking of today's younger generation of chefs is evolving, while still keeping a firm hand on traditional recipes. This strong attachment to the old way of doing things means that most people still refuse to give in to the processed foods available in supermarkets and will most likely go out of their way to get local and seasonal produce. This explains why there is no such thing as Italian food in Italy – instead there's Roman, Neapolitan, Venetian, Sicilian and so on – and what you see on a menu in Naples will be impossible to find in Venice and vice versa.

Rome is known for its four 'royal' pastas: *amatriciana*, *carbonara*, *cacio e pepe* and *gricia*. Everyone has their own little variations on these, but they all follow the same basic rules. Here are my recipes for two of my favourites. (And if any of my Roman friends are reading this, please don't kill me – this is how I like them!)

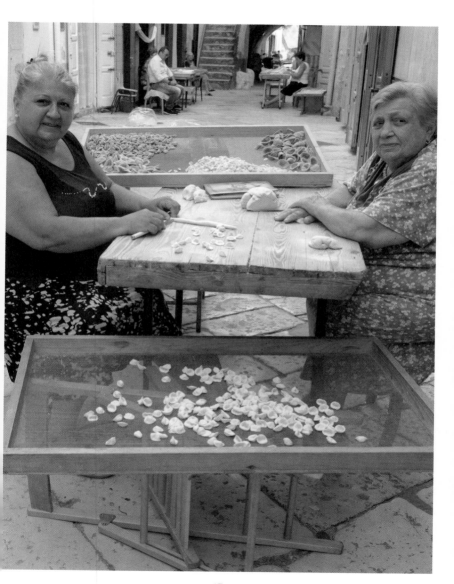

CARBONARA

The key to the perfect *carbonara* is the strategic timing when adding the raw egg to the already cooked pasta: add it when the pasta is too hot and the egg will scramble; if the pasta is too cold, you will be slurping up raw egg. You need to be patient with this dish. Try it over and over again until you perfect it – enough to make any Roman proud.

SERVES 4

500g rigatoni (this is the only acceptable shape in Rome; if you use anything else, you will start a war)

2 thick slices *guanciale*

1 whole egg and 3 egg yolks

100g Pecorino Romano or Parmigiano Reggiano (or a little of both!) plus extra to serve

black pepper

1. Heat a pan of salted water, and when it comes to the boil, throw the pasta in until perfectly al dente. (When you drain the pasta, make sure to keep a cup of the cooking water, you might need it later on.)

2. Chop the *guanciale* into thin strips and cook in a pan. You will notice it will release a lot of fat; make sure you save all of this as we use it instead of olive oil for this dish. Remove from the heat.

3. In a separate bowl, stir the whole egg and the three yolks together with the cheese and black pepper until you have a thick paste. I like to add some of the fat from the *guanciale* to this mixture. Stir well.

4. Place the cooked pasta in the pan with the pork, coating it in the fat. Remember the pan should be off the heat now (to allow the pasta to cool a little).

5. Once it is coated in fat, add the pasta to the bowl with the egg mixture. Add a little bit of the reserved pasta cooking water and stir quickly. To serve, add a sprinkle of grated cheese and some more ground black pepper.

AMATRICIANA

When people ask me what my last meal on earth would be, I always answer *amatriciana*. The mixture of the crispy *guanciale*, sweet tomato sauce and salty pecorino makes this the perfect dish for any occasion. Traditionally, we are meant to use bucatini as a pasta shape but, to be honest, they are almost impossible to eat (they can be very slippery and difficult to twirl around your fork in an orderly manner), and so I substitute them with spaghetti or rigatoni.

SERVES 4

2 thick slices *guanciale*
a generous pinch of
   hot pepper flakes
   (optional)
50ml white wine
500g tinned tomatoes
   (make sure they are
   whole, no matter
   the size)
500g rigatoni or
   spaghetti
80g grated Pecorino
   Romano

1. Heat a pan of water until boiling.
2. In the meantime, chop the *guanciale* into thin strips and place it in a hot pan with no olive oil. Let it cook on a low heat until the clear fat is released, then add the hot pepper (if using) and white wine. Continue to cook on a low heat until the wine has evaporated.
3. Remove the *guanciale* strips from the pan and set aside, making sure you leave the clear fat in the pan. Add the tomatoes and cook until thickened.
4. In the meantime, add the pasta to the boiling water and cook according to the packet instructions (or 2–3 minutes less, if you like a bite to your pasta).
5. Add the *guanciale* to the thickened sauce and cook for a further 5 minutes.
6. Drain the pasta when still very al dente, reserving a cup of the cooking water. Keep stirring until the pasta is perfectly cooked (about 1 minute). While mixing, add the grated pecorino, but keep some aside for serving.
7. To serve, plate the pasta and top with pecorino.

Fare la scarpetta

This phrase literally means 'to make the shoe' and refers to the very common practice of picking up a little piece of bread at the end of a meal, and using it to mop up all the sauce from the plate, leaving it perfectly clean: your finger acts as the 'leg' here, pushing the 'shoe' (the bread) across the plate. Most Italians will ask if something is wrong when they see someone who is not doing the *scarpetta* after eating a big bowl of pasta. It's a sign of appreciation, and it shows the host or the waiter that you thoroughly enjoyed what you ate.

SHOPPING FOR FOOD
La spesa

Traditionally in Italy, shopping for food was done by the mother of the household each and every single day. There are a few reasons for this:

Italians come from a history of war and poverty, so for years people only bought what they needed and could afford. This mentality is still deeply entrenched in their daily routine.

In cities like Rome, or in small towns, everything is within walking distance. This means that it usually only takes one hour to walk to the butcher for meat, the bakery for bread and the market for fruits and vegetables. And only buying what you need for each day means you can easily carry it home.

Apartments are not big, so most people have a small fridge which can only fit so much stuff.

Going to the supermarket and buying enough food to last a whole week is a concept that I only discovered relatively recently. For me, walking around a neighbourhood, chatting with all the different shop vendors, seeing what's in season and then bringing it all home has always felt relaxing and oddly therapeutic. Most Italians develop such strong relationships with

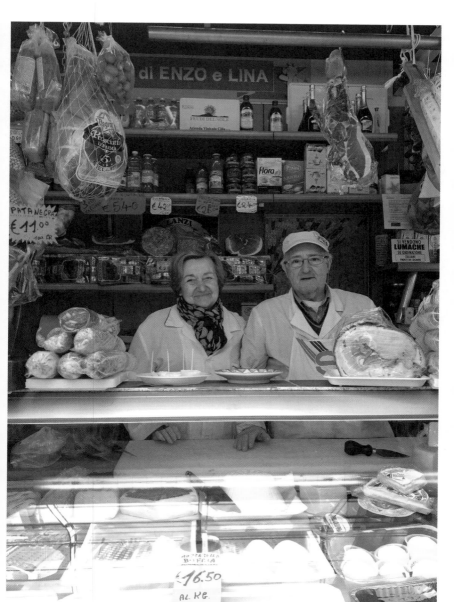

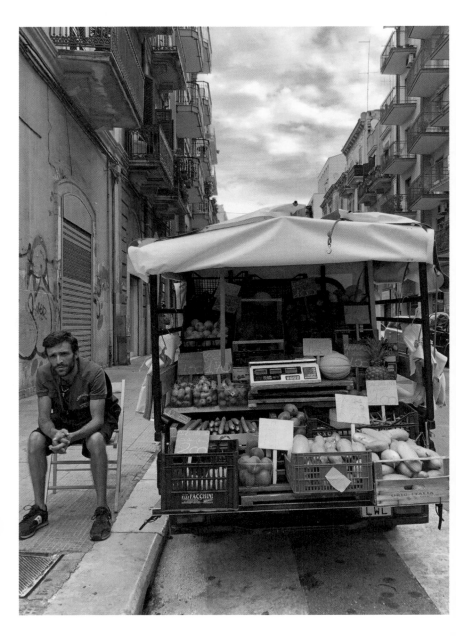

their vendors that they become like family members. They are the people they trust with their food, and the ones they see every day for years and years. Being loyal to vendors also pays off: it means getting the best produce (carefully selected for them), discounts and lots of smiles and recipe ideas. They might even get to skip the line some days.

I usually set off for the market with a clear idea of what I want to buy and later cook, but there are some days when I have no idea what I feel like. Luckily, most vendors have very strong opinions and will help me. If they know me well enough, they will actually make the decision for me as to what I should be eating for lunch or dinner that day.

When I first moved to my own apartment in Rome, I quickly created a habit of always going to the same fruit-and-vegetable vendor. One morning, I was extremely undecided on what to cook for lunch that day, but my eyes kept being drawn to the beautiful artichokes on display. Franco, my vendor, noticed that I was staring at them and made the decision that I would be eating them for lunch. I tried to explain that artichokes had always scared me – I absolutely adored the flavour, but had never mastered the art of cleaning and cooking them. That morning, Franco took me under his wing because he claimed that no Roman in their right mind should be afraid of artichokes. We sat down together and he taught me to clean them, one by one, until I'd mastered it. He then sent me home with a bag full of cleaned artichokes, a recipe scribbled on a piece of paper and a heart full of love for my dear Franco.

SHOPPING IN AN ITALIAN MARKET:
SOME DOs AND DON'Ts

Each country has a different way of doing things, and when travelling, most people can feel overwhelmed in markets – the noise, fruits and vegetables you don't recognise, people yelling things at you and, the biggest question of all: how do you ask for what you want?

Somehow, Italians manage to instinctively know how to navigate their way around any market, but here's a quick guide for everyone else:

1. **Don't touch the merchandise.** This is the most important rule. You don't get to touch what you're buying until you've paid for it. It might seem counterintuitive because how can you tell if the tomato you're buying is good if you don't pick it up? Well, you just have to assume that everything the vendor has is delicious (so you don't need to check yourself by touching). Plus, the relationship between market vendors and customers in Italy is built on mutual trust, so the longer you keep going to the same stand, the more likely that the vendor will let you pick out your own produce.

2. **Shop in season (see more below).** Italy still eats based on the seasons, so don't be frustrated if you can't find tomatoes in an Italian market in the middle of winter. Take a look around and be inspired instead by something you wouldn't normally find at home.

3. **Get your numbers right.** Finding out the prices in Italian markets can be a little confusing. Everything is priced by weight (per kilo), and if you want something, you have to ask by the gram (*etto*). For example, '*Potrei avere 2 etti di spinaci per favore?*' – 'Could I please have 200 grams of spinach?'

4. **Smile.** Italians can never resist a smile, so even if you think you have no idea what you are doing, just give them a big smile and they will help you out.

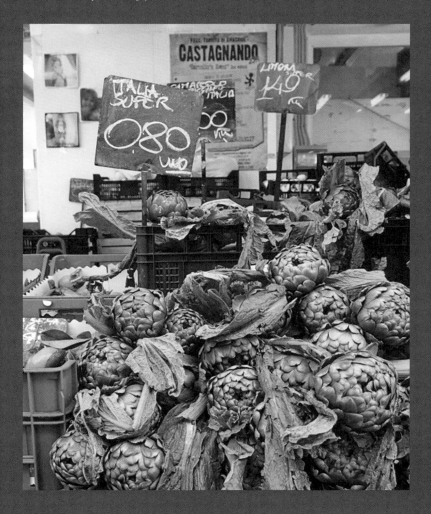

SEASONALITY
Stagionalità

For Italians, eating seasonally is a sort of comforting ritual.

I don't know about you, but the excitement of finally getting the fruit or vegetable I've been waiting for all year makes me feel like a kid unwrapping gifts at Christmas. Some are only available a few weeks a year, and some just for a few days.

Certain fruits and vegetables remind me of specific moments in my childhood and I associate each one with the things I love most in each season. Like swelteringly hot summer days, when you suddenly find yourself hanging out underneath a fig tree eating one fruit after another until you realise you're completely figged-out.

Or the sweetness of *kaki* (persimmons) that magically appear at the beginning of November and leave you wanting more at the end of the month when it's already too late. The crunchiness of *puntarelle* (chicory). In Rome, we eat so much of it we have totally overdosed by the time winter has come to an end. And then we have spring's glorious gifts: an abundance of artichokes, fava beans and fresh peas.

While we know that eating in Italy is something of a sacred activity, what makes the food so delicious is the respect for local and seasonal ingredients. When you eat seasonally, you are assured a delicious meal, filled with fruits and vegetables at the height of their flavour.

I know it's not easy for everyone to gain access to fresh local ingredients, but these days, there are more and more farmers' markets and home-delivery systems that come directly to your doorstep from farms around you. When you eat seasonally you will discover new ingredients, recipes and flavours, and you can create your own yearly rituals.

The key to eating with the seasons is patience. There are a few seasonal recipes I love and look forward to all year. Here are the ones that top my list.

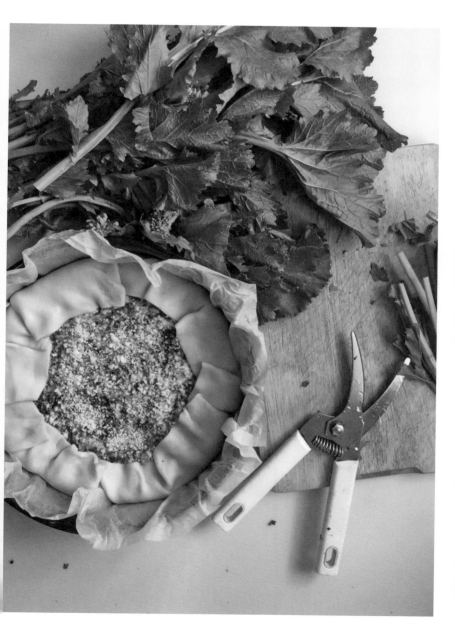

ORECCHIETTE WITH CIME DI RAPA

Orecchiette con le cime di rapa

This is something I grew up eating in my grandma's house. She would make it as a welcome dinner every time we went down to see her. This is also the first recipe she passed on to my mom, so she could cook it for her precious son (my dad). In Italy, *cime di rapa* are available in the colder months (the English equivalent is broccoli rabe; it won't taste exactly the same, but it will still be delicious!) and what I find myself doing is cooking large batches and freezing them for when they are no longer available.

SERVES 4

1kg broccoli rabe
500g orecchiette
5 anchovy fillets
　(in olive oil)
2 garlic cloves
a pinch of red pepper
　flakes

1. Wash and trim the greens. Keep the flowering heads and tender parts and remove any that are too tough (usually the very ends of the stem).
2. Heat a pan of salted water. Once boiling, add the orecchiette and cook for about 5 minutes. Throw in the broccoli and cook together for about a total of 12 minutes.
3. In the meantime, chop the anchovies and garlic and add them to a pan with the olive oil from the anchovies. Heat until the garlic turns golden and the anchovies melt. Remove from the heat.
4. Once the pasta and broccoli is cooked, drain saving a cup of the cooking water. Return the pan with anchovies to a low heat and add the pasta. Stir together until the pasta has absorbed all the olive oil. If it seems too dry, you can add some of the reserved cooking water.
5. To serve, sprinkle with red pepper flakes.

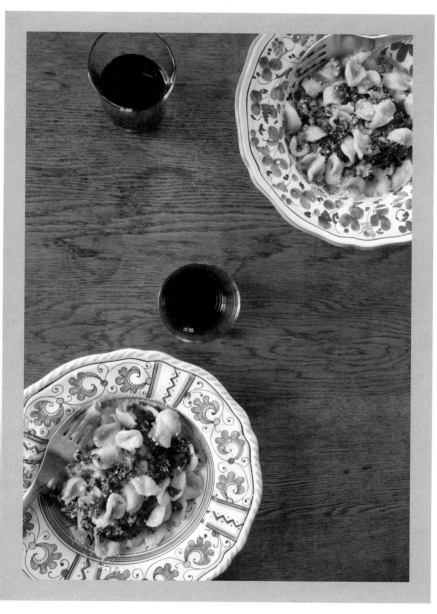

FENNEL AND ORANGE SALAD
Insalata di finocchi e arance

These days, with food being shipped all over the world, people tend to forget that oranges actually have a season. We are so used to seeing them in every supermarket, year-round, that we forget how a delicious orange in season can actually taste like pure sunshine. This is what I make when I am tired of eating heavier, warm winter foods, and feel like eating something that reminds me of summer in the dead of winter. (Both oranges and fennel are winter foods, even though this feels like a 'summery' dish.) It's also very quick, so it's my go-to when I don't have a lot of time.

SERVES 4

3 whole fennel bulbs
2 oranges
black olives
   (as bitter and
   salty as possible)
juice of 1 lemon
olive oil (as much
   as you like, you
   can never have
   too much!)
salt and pepper

1. Wash, dry and trim the fennel and cut into medium-to-thin slices. Place on a flat platter.
2. Remove both ends of the oranges. With a knife, take the rest of the peel off, making sure you remove all the white parts. Cut into thin slices, starting from either end (you should get perfectly round slices). Save as much of the juice released from the orange as possible (it will be good for the dressing).
3. Place the oranges and olives on top of the fennel (you can remove the pits from the olives beforehand).
4. Drizzle some of the reserved orange juice and the lemon juice, olive oil, salt and plenty of ground black pepper over the top. Mix it all up just before serving.

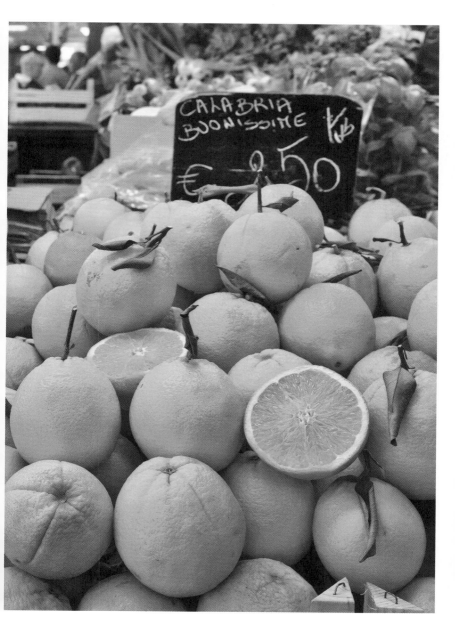

VEGETABLES FROM 'THE VINE'
Vignarola

When spring arrives, we are blessed with an abundance of delicious vegetables. This is a Roman side dish (I also like it as a main) that makes use of the delights that spring has to offer.

SERVES 4

500g fresh peas
500g fresh fava beans
500g artichokes
250g spring onions
100g *guanciale*
olive oil (enough to
   cover your entire pan,
   you should have a
   generous layer)
salt and pepper
1 small bunch mint

1. Prepare all the ingredients (except the mint): remove both the peas and the fava beans from their pods (reserving the pods). Clean and cut the artichokes into quarters (see p.64). Save the stalks and add them along with the artichokes to a bowl with water and lemon juice to prevent them from oxidising. Chop the onions, removing the green parts. Cut the *guanciale* into thin strips.

2. Add the scraps of all the vegetables (pea and fava bean pods and the green onion stalks) to a small pot of boiling water to make a quick vegetable broth.

3. Grab a pan and pour in the olive oil. Add the *guanciale* strips and cook until crispy. Then add the onion until softened.

4. Add the artichokes to the pan, along with a ladle of the vegetable broth. Cover and cook for about 5 minutes. Add the peas and favas and cook for a further 10 minutes, along with an additional ladle of broth.

5. Once all the vegetables seem cooked, add the mint (you should chop this at the very last minute, so it stays fresh), salt and pepper.

FRIED COURGETTES WITH MINT AND VINEGAR

Zucchine alla scapece

Courgettes are one of my favourite vegetables, but they can sometimes be bland and watery. This recipe makes them irresistible though! In the autumn, when courgettes are no longer available, I've also had pumpkin cooked this way, and it was absolutely delicious, so feel free to play around with other vegetables.

SERVES 4

1 litre vegetable oil
7 small courgettes
1 garlic clove
80ml white wine
  vinegar
salt and pepper
chopped fresh mint
  (about 4 tbsp)

1. Add the vegetable oil to a medium (high-sided) pan over a medium heat, ensuring the oil does not go more than halfway up the pot.

2. While you wait for the oil to reach the required temperature (177°C), slice the courgettes into medium to thick discs. In a bowl, pound the garlic and mix it with the vinegar, salt and ground black pepper (to taste).

3. When the oil has reached the right temperature, lower about a third of the courgette slices into it for about 2 or 3 minutes, until golden. Remove with a slotted spoon and place them on a plate lined with kitchen paper to absorb any excess oil. Repeat with the remaining courgette slices until they are all fried. Sprinkle with salt.

4. Leave the courgettes to cool before tossing them in a bowl with the garlicky vinegar and mint. Add more salt if needed. Allow to marinate for a couple of hours before eating.

HOW TO CLEAN ARTICHOKES

In rome, artichokes are considered the holy figure of all vegetables.
We wait all year for their season, and once they are available we eat them every day until they are gone again. Eating them is easy, but cleaning them can be somewhat tricky. With these simple instructions and a little practice, I am positive you will master the art of artichoke cleaning in no time.

1. Artichokes oxidize quickly, which turns them brown, so before you start, fill a bowl with cold water and squeeze half a lemon into it. Use the other half of the lemon to rub all the visible artichoke surfaces and then place the artichokes in the lemon water until you are ready to cook with them.

2. Break off the tough, outer leaves of each artichoke, until you get down to the leaves which are tender. You'll know you're getting to the tender part by the colour; they are usually yellow on the bottom third and pale violet at the top. When you break off the leaves try to leave on as much of the root of the leaf as possible.

3. Once you have taken off the tough outer leaves, use a small knife to gently trim away the bright green parts from the stem end. Don't cut off too much, just the green part. This section is quite bitter. Immediately rub the cut part with lemon.

4. Turn the artichoke on its side and cut off the top third (the pointy end of the artichoke). Make sure your knife is really sharp. Immediately rub the cut part with lemon and replace in the lemon water.

5. In Rome, the choke (the centre fuzzy part) is edible, but if it seems too prickly and tough, then remove it by scooping it out with the edge of the knife.

6. Don't forget the stem – it's my favourite part! Just remove the outer layer with your knife, the rest is completely edible and tender.

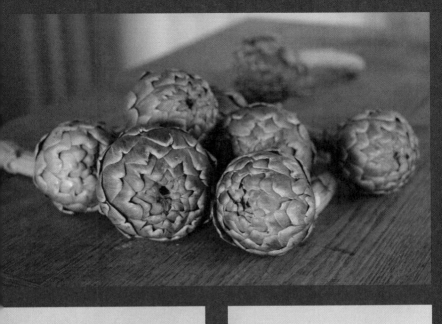

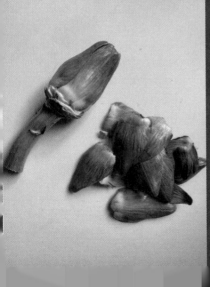

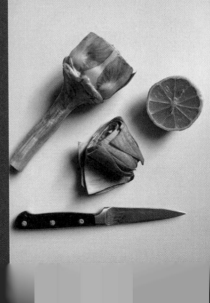

DRIED AND FRESH PASTA
Pasta asciutta e pasta fresca

One of the questions I'm most commonly asked is: 'What is the difference between fresh and dried pasta?' This is usually followed by, 'Is fresh pasta better?'

In my eyes they are all glorious creations, put on this earth to make us happy. I also think they shouldn't be compared: they are made with different ingredients and different methods, so are two very different things. Here are a few facts about pasta:

Dried pasta

This used to be a lot more common in southern Italy but has now become popular all over the country. The reason for its popularity in the south is mainly that it uses durum wheat, which used to be grown only in that region. Also, that part of the country had (and still has) the perfect weather conditions to dry the pasta naturally, out in the open air. Today, because of hygiene regulations, all pasta must be dried indoors. And this is where the big difference comes in between dried pasta brands: big industrial brands power-dry their pasta very quickly to make as much as possible in a shorter time. This means that when you cook that pasta, it will never be the perfect consistency and will most likely fall apart. High-quality dried pasta takes a lot longer to dry (hence the difference in price). This also means it needs a much longer cooking time, and the pasta will be perfectly al dente. Dried pasta also comes in over 350 different shapes which cannot be matched by the fresh version, and has a rougher surface for all the delicious sauces to stick to.

Fresh pasta

Even though I grew up eating a lot more dried pasta (that's just what people in Rome eat), I associate fresh pasta with the purest form of unconditional

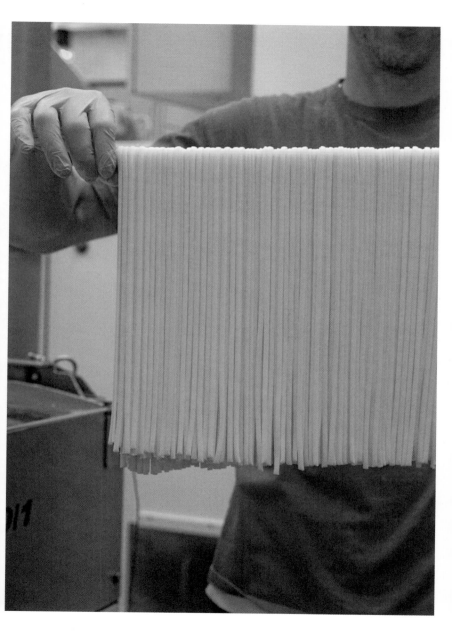

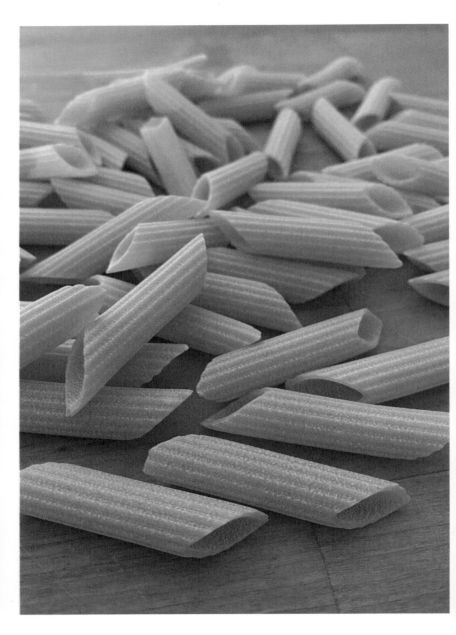

love. Mothers and grandmas all over the country take time to slowly prepare their favourite shapes, so they can feed friends and family. It's also associated with the good times: Sunday lunches, Christmas, religious celebrations and weddings.

Fresh pasta is made with eggs, strong flour and water. Because of the eggs, it has a very short shelf life and is best eaten the day it is made. The eggs also give it a much softer, yet chewy consistency, so it pairs much better with some sauces than others. For example, a rich tomato sauce with meat will go better with a fresh pasta, while a light seafood one will go very well with a dried pasta.

So how do you choose?

For fresh pasta, all you need is really good eggs and enough time and patience on your hands. When it comes to dried pasta, you have to make sure you are getting the best there is, even if it means importing it directly from Italy. I can still remember the day I ate my first bowl of high-quality dried pasta as a seven-year-old: it changed my life for ever, and I will never forget the feeling of pure joy when taking that first bite.

HERE ARE SOME OF MY FAVOURITE BRANDS OF ARTISANAL PASTA. GIVE THEM A TRY – THEY ARE ALL AVAILABLE ONLINE:

Benedetto Cavalieri
Rustichella
Gentile
Martelli
Felicetti

PASTA SHAPES

As a small kid, when we spent summer mornings at our babysitter's home, my favourite time of day was when her mother, Sandra, announced it was time to choose the pasta shape for lunch. My sister and I would run to the kitchen, since the first one there got to choose. Of course, we would end up screaming and fighting because I always wanted the *lumache* and she wanted the penne. The result? Poor Sandra had to cook two different kinds of pasta every day for lunch to keep us both happy and well fed.

A LITTLE GUIDE TO PASTA SHAPES

Italy is home to thousands of different pasta shapes, from classic spaghetti to unusual shapes handmade in the various regions. Here are six of my personal favourites:

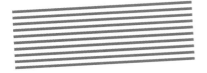 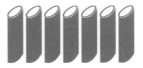

SPAGHETTI
Probably one of the most famous (and loved) shapes worldwide, there is something oddly romantic and satisfying about twirling these luscious noodles around your fork. I love them with a simple tomato sauce or even with no sauce at all, just some *aglio, olio e peperoncino* (garlic, olive oil and hot pepper).

RIGATONI
This is Rome's favourite pasta shape: the thick consistency tastes great al dente, and is perfect for *carbonara* and *amatriciana*. It's a simple shape that makes everyone happy, so I always have at least a few packs in my pantry.

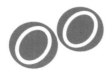

ORECCHIETTE

Originally from the region of Puglia, I love *orecchiette con cime di rapa* (with broccoli rabe, see recipe page 58). The vegetables fall apart and perfectly coat the pasta along with anchovies, olive oil and garlic.

FARFALLE

Another pasta shape that reminds me of my childhood, especially those long summer days spent at the beach. Farfalle pair great with cold ingredients like cherry tomatoes, mozzarella and basil, and make an exceptional *pasta fredda* (pasta salad).

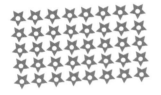

PASTINA

These tiny little specks of pasta are perfect for a cold winter day when you crave some delicious homemade broth. Kids love it (it reminds me of my childhood) and don't forget to drizzle it with a lot of freshly grated parmigiano before serving.

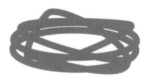

FRESH TAGLIATELLE

I had to include a fresh pasta, and this is what comes to mind when I think of a special meal like Sunday lunch, Christmas or Easter. The soft texture pairs well with a rich bolognese but also works well with something more creamy-cheesy.

PIZZA NIGHT

Another food that has popularised Italian cuisine worldwide is pizza, and one of the most sacred evenings in an Italian household is 'pizza night'. This is usually on a Sunday, most likely because somebody from the family will have spent half the day cooking up a feast and does not feel like cooking again the same evening. Also, with Sunday lunch being a richer meal than usual (see p. 42), people can crave something lighter and quick, like pizza, for dinner (yes, pizza is considered light in Italy). Sunday night is also when other types of restaurants are often closed, so it gives those owners a chance to have a break and eat a pizza themselves.

Sunday is a day for rest, and when I think of Dolce Far Niente, one of the first things that comes to mind is pizza night. A chance to rest from your job, from housework, from eating the healthier food options you've had during the week. It's a casual, happy and fun evening, and all you need to focus on is the pizza and the company right in front of you.

Growing up, we would spend every Sunday night at the same neighbourhood pizza joint, and we would find ourselves sitting right next to all the non-pizza restaurant owners from the neighbourhood. Pizza night is also a chance to have a beer or fizzy drink, since Italians believe these carbonated beverages will complement the pizza.

Pizza night always starts with a mixture of fried items to share between the whole table. Fried food varies all over Italy, but the most popular ones in Rome are *suppli* (little balls of rice cooked with tomato sauce and mozzarella, then fried), *fiore di zucca* (my absolute favourite – a courgette flower stuffed with melted mozzarella and an anchovy) and *baccalà* (the Italian version of fish and chips, a fried fillet of salt cod). After that, everyone gets their own pizza; we never split one in half and it never comes pre-sliced. Once you have cut the pizza, it's ok to 'exchange' a few slices with other people at the table, in order to try different varieties. It's also ok to pick up the slices with your hands; it's the only way to truly enjoy pizza and get the perfect bite!

Remember to keep it simple with the ingredients: most Italians prefer to order an ordinary *margherita* (tomato, mozzarella and basil) or *marinara* (tomato, garlic and oregano), keeping pizza night light, as intended.

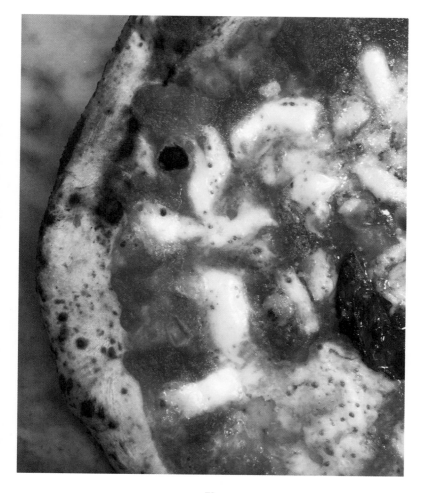

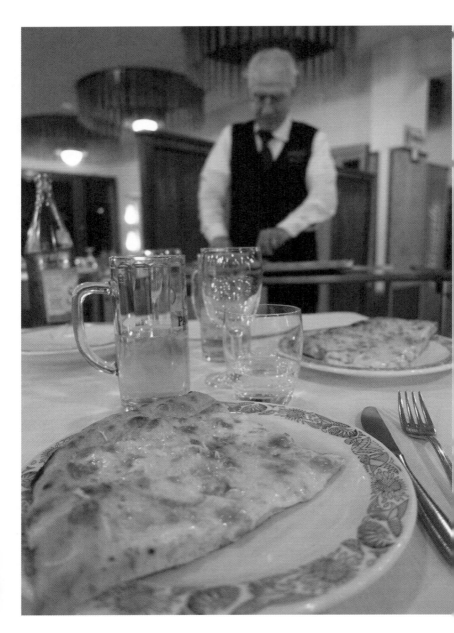

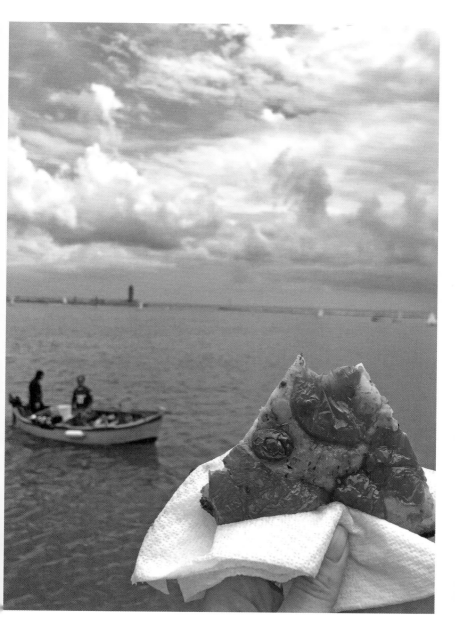

WINE
Vino

Even though the drinking age in Italy was raised to eighteen in 2012 (it was sixteen before that, and further back still there was no restriction), young Italians learn all there is to know about alcohol consumption at home. Wine has always been part of the table setting, and from a very young age Italians learn to sip and enjoy it as an accompaniment to their food. This means you will rarely see young Italians binge drinking or getting drunk because it is no big deal to them to have access to alcohol – it's simply what they have at home with their parents at meals.

Since wine is meant to pair well with the food you are eating, most table wines in restaurants are surprisingly not bad, usually using local grapes and at a very fair price. The same generally goes for everyday wine used at home.

Consuming alcohol in Italy completely revolves around food: you are either drinking to accompany a meal or you are given free snacks when sipping a cocktail at a bar.

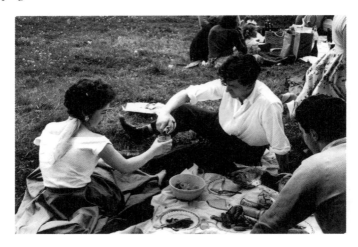

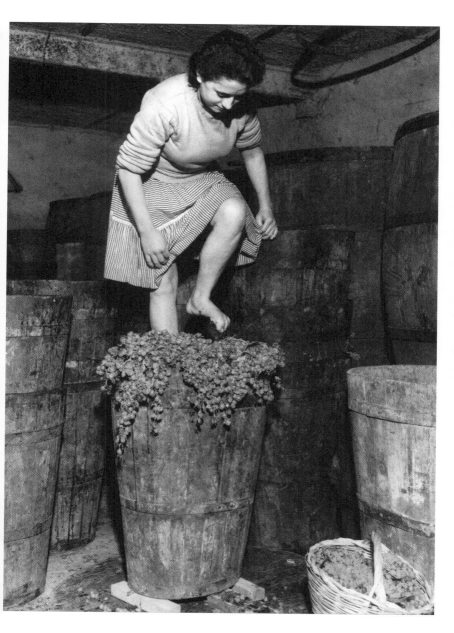

DIGESTION
Digestione

While Italians seemingly eat all the time, they are also extremely attentive to the way they eat. After eating good food, the second-most important thing in Italy is having 'good' digestion. But when speaking about digestion in Italy, it is not necessarily about the whole 'digestive process'. Rather, it's the settling of the stomach thanks to a combination of the right foods, eaten at the right time, in the right place and at the right temperature. Meeting these requirements will ensure a perfectly healthy digestion.

When talking about proper digestion, Italians' worst enemy (and fear) is the cold. According to them, a cold drink can completely block and quite literally 'freeze' your digestion. After a workout, chugging a bottle of ice-cold water supposedly equals immediate death in this country. Another factor that could negatively impact proper digestion, they say, is time. In order for food to settle properly, you need to eat it without feeling rushed, taking all the time you need. I've met people in Italy who would rather not eat at all than eat while being rushed.

After meals, you can aid your digestion with a drink referred to as a *digestivo*. Most commonly, this is *amaro*, a bitter, herb-infused liqueur, and every region of Italy has its own recipe, based on whatever roots, herbs and fruits are grown locally.

Another thing which leads to immediate death (according to most Italian grandmas) happens during the summer months, and especially affects kids on the beach. After eating their lunch, they are not allowed into the water for at least two hours (giving them enough time to digest properly). This is why if you find yourself on an Italian beach around lunchtime, you will see very few people in the water (especially not kids). Most likely they will be napping on their beach chairs in the shade instead. Since I grew up with an American mother, this rule never applied to me. I can still remember the jealousy of all the other kids at the beach because I was allowed to swim right after lunch and, by some miracle, I survived. Even after these kids used me as an example, their mothers would not budge: no swimming for at least two hours after eating. End of story.

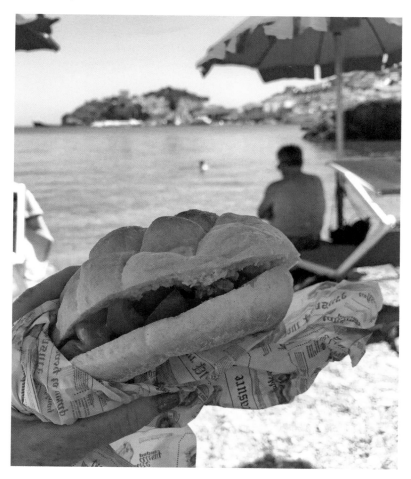

ITALIAN DINING ETIQUETTE
Come mangiare all'Italiana

The most holy room in an Italian home is the kitchen, which is usually where the dining table is and, therefore, where families reunite every day, for lunch and dinner. This is where an Italian family talks (and they talk a lot) – about life, work, education, expenses, food and holidays. This is also where children start their education. Because from a very young age, they do as the grown-ups do. Kids eat whatever was cooked for everyone else and they sit, talk, use a knife and fork and only get up when they have eaten everything on the plate.

Here are a few 'rules' that Italians learn as kids when sitting down at the dinner table:

1

To cheese or not to cheese?

Italians can often be quite strict with their food rules, especially when it comes to adding cheese to pasta. For some pastas or rice dishes, it can be seen as sacrilege to add extra cheese (usually anything with seafood because the strong flavour of grated parmigiano or pecorino will completely overpower the dish). Another big no-no is adding grated cheese to pasta dishes with truffles or mushrooms (for the same reason).

2

Bread

An Italian table is not complete without a bread basket placed right in the middle. However, there are a lot of misconceptions around that bread basket. In all my years eating out in Italy, I've noticed that some people (usually tourists) go straight for the bread basket, eating all the bread before the menu has even arrived. In Italy, bread is not meant to be eaten before the rest of the food is on the table, but only during the meal. It's there to accompany the

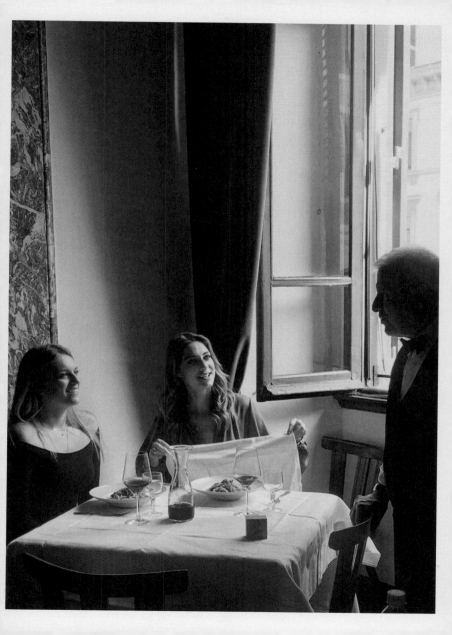

food, not as a starter. Dipping bread in olive oil before the meal starts? You will never see an Italian doing that. And if you think about it, why would you want to fill up on bread before the food has come? How are you going to enjoy all the delicious starters, pastas and meats? Save room for all the amazingness that is about to come.

3
Cin cin – cheers!

When everyone has a full plate of food in front of them, that is when Italians usually raise their glasses and toast. However, like everything food-related in Italy, there are rules, and most of them have to do with superstition:

- You are only allowed to toast if your glass if filled with an alcoholic beverage (usually wine or beer). If you don't drink alcohol, pour a little of it in your glass just for the cheering; it's considered very bad luck to toast with water.

- Never cross arms with other people at the table. Again, this is very bad luck, and Italians take their superstitions very seriously indeed.

- Most important of all: always lock eyes with the person you are toasting with. If you don't look right into their eyes, it's a sign that you are most likely a traitor. This goes back to the Middle Ages when it was common for people to place poison in their enemies' drinks and food. So by looking the other person in the eye, you are assuring them that the drink is poison-free. Today, it's not about the poison (those times are thankfully long gone), but more about maintaining traditions.

4
Salad

As touched on earlier (see p. 42), (see p. 42) salad is never served as a starter, but as a side dish to your main course (meat or fish). You will notice it will never come pre-dressed, but you will find some olive oil, salt and white wine vinegar on the table. This is for you to dress your own salad. Italians believe that eating a fresh green salad simply dressed with olive oil and vinegar at the end of your meal with help to cleanse the palate and aid digestion (it's always about digestion!).

5

Don't cut your pasta

Twirl, twirl and twirl! Long pasta is long for a reason, and that reason is because it's meant to twirl entirely around your fork, creating the perfect mess-free bite. The secret is to cook the pasta to perfection and to have the right pasta-to-sauce ratio (there should be plenty of sauce, but not so much that your pasta is swimming in it), in order to allow the spaghetti to stay in place when twirling them around your fork. Learning to whirl your luscious spaghetti perfectly around your fork can be fun, so why not

take it slow one evening and perfect the art? In certain parts of Italy, people use spoons to help with the twirling process, but not in Rome! Here, it's seen as a weakness and no one would dream of using one. The trick is starting from the edge of the plate, twirling and moving the pasta towards you until you have created the perfect mess-free bite which should perfectly fit into your mouth.

6

Wine or water

Just as the bread basket is mandatory, bottles of wine and water are too. Neither is ever missing from an Italian table and they are the only acceptable drinks to accompany your meal. Anything else is believed to mess with the flavours of the food. The one exception, as I mentioned earlier, is pizza night (see p. 72), when soft beverages and beer are 100 per cent acceptable.

WATCH WHAT YOU SAY WHEN YOU TALK ABOUT ITALIAN FOOD

To get an idea of just how dangerous it is to offend an Italian over food, try looking up 'Italian' recipes (traditional Italian recipes cooked by non-Italian chefs) online and have a good laugh while reading the comments. There are also Twitter accounts, like 'Italians mad at food', where you can experience the wrath of Italians as it is incited by affronts to their cuisine. I've seen countless fights in Italy over the correct way of making dishes like *carbonara* – small details like the choice between pecorino or parmigiano, pancetta or *guanciale*, long pasta or short. But when Italians come face to face with the way people cook up this recipe abroad, it's as if they've been punched in the heart. Chicken instead of pork? Addition of heavy cream? Parsley and onions? Italians are ok with people cooking whatever they like, but please don't call it a *carbonara* in front of them (unless you want to experience a full-on Italian pasta rage).

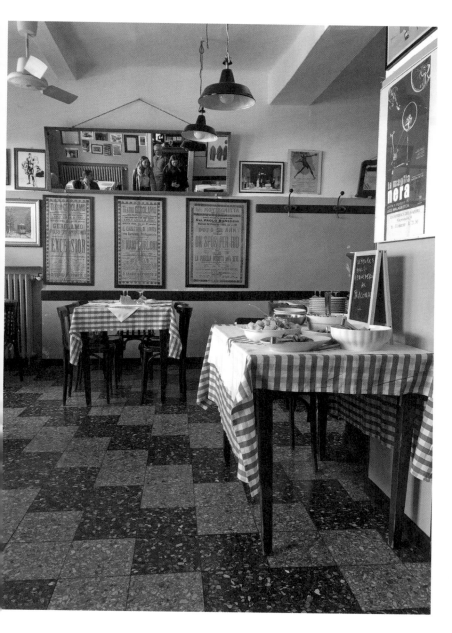

THE ITALIAN KITCHEN AND PANTRY

La cucina e la dispensa

The most important room in an Italian home is the kitchen. It is usually where the TV is, where you sit down to eat or to have coffee, where food is constantly on the stove and where the mamma – and all those who follow her – hangs out.

Italian homes are extremely clean and well organised. After each meal is cooked, the kitchen is scrubbed to perfection. Without a doubt, it is considered the beating heart of any Italian home, and so must always appear perfect (you never know when a guest or neighbour might pop over). Because spaces are so small in Italy, most people will not have a formal dining room to accommodate guests, but usually a smaller table right in the middle of the kitchen. It's the room where family and friends get together. And it's also the warmest room in the house because there is always something cooking. If Dolce Far Niente had to be associated with a room, it would be the kitchen.

Whenever I am in somebody else's home, I love peeking into their pantry or cupboards. Even though you can create amazing feasts that include meat, fish and vegetables from the market, some of the very best meals are those made using whatever you find in your pantry, without even leaving the house. And this usually means pasta.

Take a look at the list on the next page and see how many of these items you can already check off your pantry and fridge list, then consider stocking up the Italian way with those that are missing, so you are always ready to cook up a meal for your loved ones.

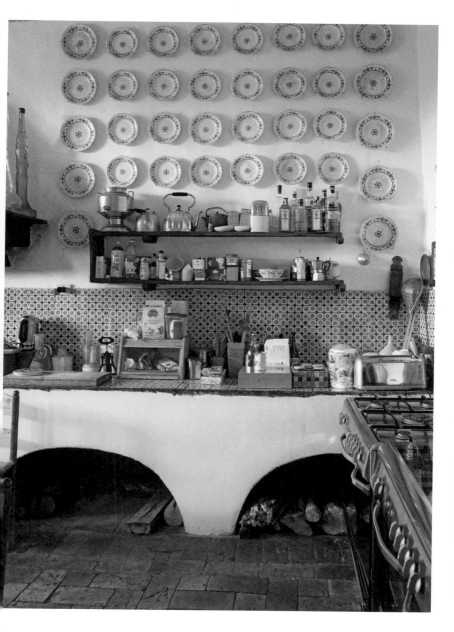

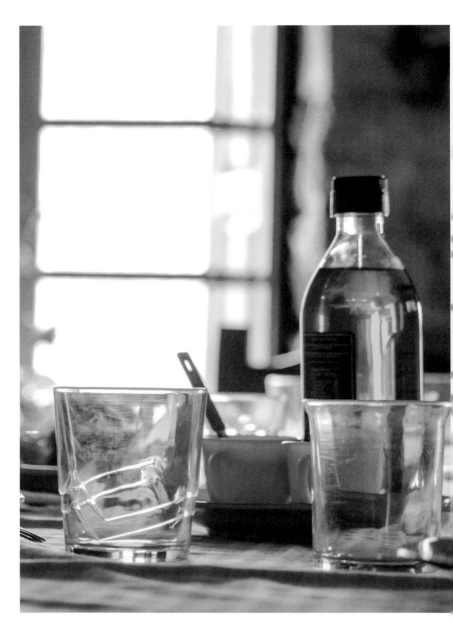

STAPLES IN AN ITALIAN PANTRY/FRIDGE

Dried pasta (Pantry)

This is the one thing you will find in every single home in Italy. The trick is to keep an array of shapes and sizes in stock. You should try to buy only high-quality dried pasta: it will change your life.

Parmigiano or Pecorino (Fridge)

A big wedge of either of these aged cheeses is all you need (or both – even better).

Guanciale (Fridge)

As a true Roman, I always have a big chunk of *guanciale* – cured pork cheek – ready to cut into delicious little cubes or strips.

Olive Oil (Pantry)

The base to everything in Italy. Don't be shy when using it. Remember to really make an effort to find the best olive oil out there, whether that means visiting a producer in Italy or getting in touch with an importer in the UK.

Canned Tomatoes (Pantry)

Whether it's passata or whole tomatoes, this is summer in a tin.

Anchovies (Pantry then fridge after opening)

I cannot stress how important a jar of high-quality anchovies is. I go through at least one every two weeks. You can add them to pasta, but also to most vegetables. I love anchovies on everything!

Peperoncino (Pantry)

Hot pepper is a perfect addition to any pasta dish. I usually have dry flakes as well as flakes preserved in olive oil.

Capers (Pantry)

These pungent, briny, tart little spheres are perfect to enhance any sauce, garnish or spread.

HOW CAN I INCORPORATE SOME OF THESE CONCEPTS INTO MY LIFE?

Food is possibly the easiest way to absorb (literally) the concept of Dolce Far Niente. In all my years of eating around Italian tables, I don't think I've ever felt rushed during a meal. Whether in northern or southern Italy, in the city or in the countryside, lunch or dinner, a meal is meant to be enjoyed as slowly as possible.

Here are some ways in which you can bring Dolce Far Niente into your own life through food:

1

Eat more pasta

Somehow pasta has been completely demonised when talking about weight loss and diets. But in Italy pasta is not the enemy, and eating it every day is the only diet they know.

Eaten in moderation, pasta can actually be good for you, but in Italy it's so much more than a source of calories and carbohydrates; it's family, it's lunch breaks and it's the closest thing to love (for me). Cooking up a plate of pasta for someone else is also a great sign of love. In Italy, one of the best ways to let someone know you care for them

is to cook food for them (whether pasta or something else), because it shows that you took the time and effort to leave them feeling full and happy. If somebody makes me a plate of delicious pasta, I instantly fall in love.

Try bringing joy to your life the Italian way by incorporating some pasta into your weekly diet. We only live once and so we should also enjoy life through the food that makes us happy. It might be a little too much to adopt the Italian lunch tradition of eating pasta every day, but maybe try doing it twice a week? As we've seen, a big part of Dolce Far Niente in Italy is sitting down for a meal, and just enjoying the food that is in front of

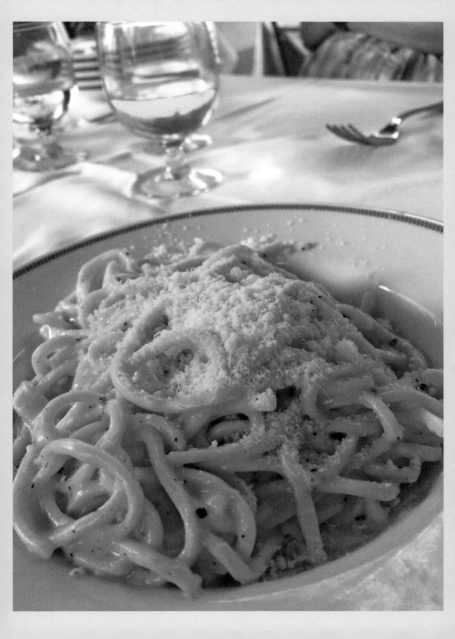

you and brings you joy. When we eat our favourite foods, we tend to feel happier and more relaxed.

2

Try cooking with the seasons

With the rise of supermarkets, we have become so accustomed to finding anything we want, at any time of the year. And when we can't find what we want, a feeling of anxiousness and despair pervades us. Try instead going back to the way things used to be (and still are in many countries): do a little online research and print out a 'what's-in-season' produce calendar. Then tape it to a wall in your house and see if you can eat with the seasons. It's a fun challenge, connects you to the earth and might lead to you discovering new fruits and vegetables to play around with in your recipes. If you can, try making a weekly stop at your local farmers' market and chat with the vendors about any produce you don't recognise and perhaps some recipes that use it. Even better, go to the market without a shopping list or a fixed idea of what you want to cook and see what you come home with.

3

Make shopping fun

Shopping for food shouldn't be a chore. Think of it as a fun activity and a way to shut your brain off from all the stress that comes along with life and work. For Italians, shopping for food is a way to get out of the house or office, be outdoors and socialise with sellers from the neighbourhood. Create your own network of vendors by building a relationship with each one of them; getting to know them will make your shopping experience a more exciting and sociable event.

4

Look up old recipes

Are there recipes you remember from your childhood? Maybe something your mum or grandma used to cook for you? Something you would always order at your preferred restaurant no matter what? Or a favourite from that summer holiday way back when with your friends? Think back to some of those dishes and try recreating them in your home (it's ok if they are not an exact replica). Thinking about them will conjure up happy memories and eating them once more will bring those memories to life.

5

Eat with family or friends

We've all done it – found ourselves running late to an appointment with no time to sit down and eat. So we grab something that we can eat on the go and call it a meal,

and while this might fill our bellies momentarily, it does very little for our overall physical and mental health. When we eat together, however, our brains receive the message that we are safe and happy, so filling our bodies with positive hormones and emotions. What's more, eating in company also benefits our health. When we eat alone, we usually eat something fast and filling, but when we are in company, studies show that we eat slower and more healthily. Put simply: eating together with family and friends can boost your mood.

6

Create your own Sunday tradition

Sunday is Italians' day to be lazy and to indulge; after all, you only live once! One Sunday a month, make your own special *pranzo della Domenica* and invite your friends and family over to share the meal. Enjoy four different courses and drink plenty of wine along with

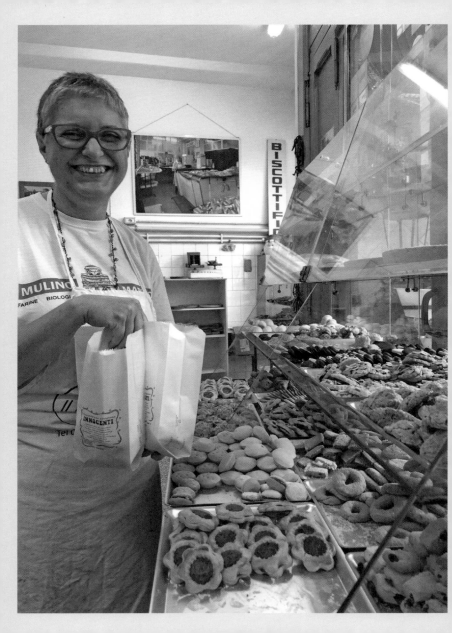

them. See how long you can manage to sit at the table for, eating and laughing (my personal record is four and a half hours).

7

Have a real lunch break

We often rush through our working day, waiting for the clock to tell us when it's time to go home. But what if we tried to make it a little more pleasant? A great way to do this is by taking a full lunch break, ideally around 60 minutes. I know this is not possible for everyone, but the effects, if you can do it, are amazing! When you leave your desk for a full lunch hour your brain will feel refreshed, and you won't have that feeling of fogginess and exhaustion in the afternoon. The result? You will be able to accomplish more during the rest of the day. Stepping away from your desk also has physical benefits: when you gobble down a meal in front of your computer it doesn't allow you to digest properly. But by taking your time and perhaps taking a short walk after your meal, you are allowing your system to process your food effectively. Think of your lunch break as an act of self-care and you will be rewarded by feeling happy, healthy and refreshed.

8

Stock up your pantry

Key to successful eating with family and friends on a regular basis is ensuring you have a well-stocked pantry. This will make the process of cooking for a group less stressful and more fun. Not only that, but it will also save you time (you won't have to rush to the shops at the last minute) and money (most pantry items last a long time). As mentioned before, cooking a meal for someone is considered a major sign of love and affection. Pleasing your family and neighbours with home-cooked food is an intrinsic part of Dolce Far Niente. It takes time, care and patience, all of which are rewarded by the smile on a guest's face when they taste their first bite.

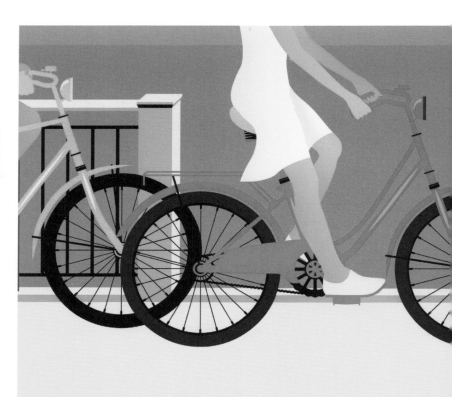

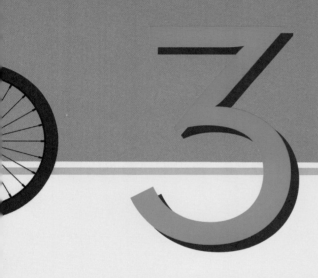

3

FAMILY &
FRIENDS

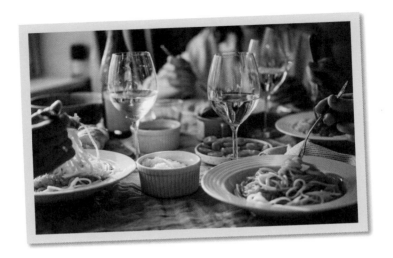

FAMILY & FRIENDS

La famiglia e gli amici

ITALIANS CAN DIFFER CONSIDERABLY FROM ONE
REGION TO THE NEXT, BUT SOMETHING THAT
TIES THEM ALL TOGETHER IS THEIR ABSOLUTE
ADORATION AND RESPECT FOR FAMILY.

Integral to every Italian's life, it not only provides economic and emotional
support, but also forms the basis of their social circle. Sure, modern Italian
families are very different from what they used to be, with fewer children,
divorce more commonplace and women more frequently now in the
workplace. But Family, with a capital 'F', still remains central to every Italian
person's sense of self. Even in a wider political context, what other languages
refer to as a 'household', Italian politicians refer to as '*la famiglia*'.

Friendships too are extremely important. Because both my parents' immediate families lived far from Rome when I was growing up, when I needed support from somebody who wasn't my parents, I would turn to my closest friends. To this day, my inner circle comprises the people I met during my earliest years at school. Maintaining the same friendships throughout the various phases of my life to date has taught me some of the most valuable lessons I needed to survive: trust, forgiveness, reliability, support, love, happiness and sacrifice. Italians don't take friendship lightly; a good friend is seen as the equivalent of an immediate family member. They are there to console you in bad times and are the makers of the happiest of times.

From a health point of view too, research has shown that Italians live longer thanks to constant social interactions and a sense of purpose.

In this chapter, I will talk about how the Italian home is formed, and what actually 'makes' the home a home, what it's like to grow old in Italy and how Italians manage to maintain meaningful friendships for their whole lives. When I talk about the 'home', I also mean family. In Italy, they are synonymous. If you think about it, the place you call home is usually where your family is, so it makes sense, right?

HOME
La casa

Nowhere is the Italian attachment to family more visible than in their living situations. While Americans and Northern Europeans usually leave home around the time of university, Italians tend to live at home with their parents until they have a real reason to leave. And 'a real reason' usually means forming their own independent family through marriage. This is partly due to economics: most grown children won't have the money to move out as soon as they finish college or high school and so they usually stay at home with their parents, often up to the age of thirty or thirty-five. And those who decide to pursue a university education generally study in their home town, so they can live at home too (even if they manage to find a part-time job while studying, they don't earn enough money to support a rent in another city, so staying at home with their parents is the logical solution). Also, living at home with their parents is an assurance of delicious food and clean laundry.

My story is slightly different in that although I was born and raised in the same tiny apartment in Rome until the age of twenty, I found my independence when I decided to move to London for college. Up until about twenty years ago, the idea of an Italian girl setting off on her own like this was seen as strange, but today things are changing and it is becoming more common, and so the traditional concept of family is slowly being moulded into something different. More and more people are leaving their home towns in search of a better education or job, usually returning when it's time to settle and build their own families.

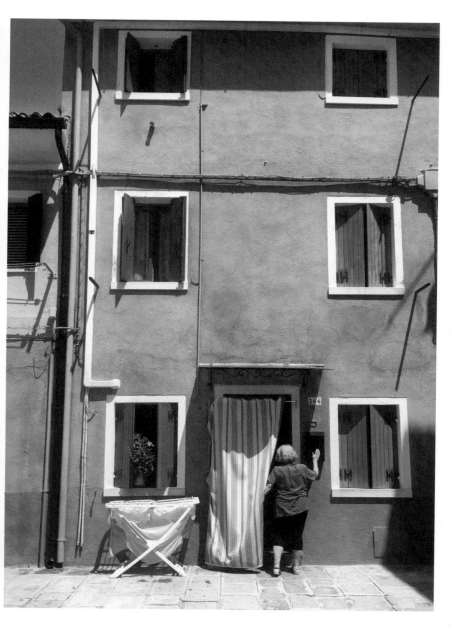

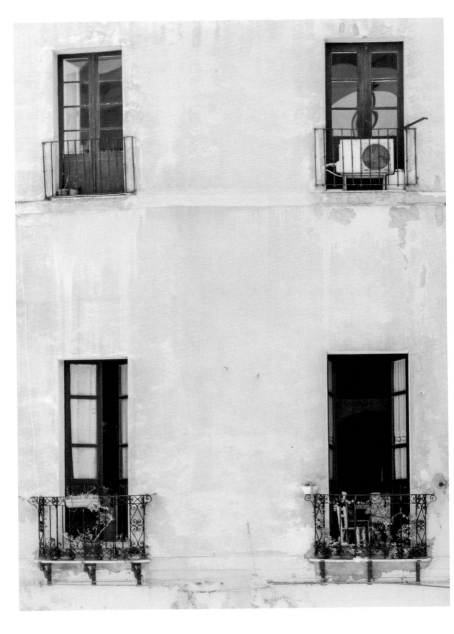

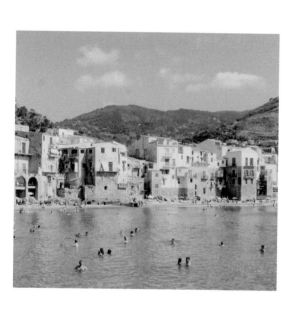

THE MOTHER
La Mamma

'La Mamma' is seen as a holy figure. Both boys and girls speak to their mothers at least three or four times a day (it's probably the most common use for mobiles in Italy). This is not to say that other cultures don't attach enough importance to their mothers, but for some reason, in Italy they are put on the highest of pedestals. Especially when it comes to their sons: Italian men have always been (and still are) in complete awe of their mothers.

To this day, while girls tend to follow in their mothers' footsteps and make an effort to learn to clean and cook, boys are not expected to master any of these life skills. That's how the term '*mammone*' – meaning 'momma's boy' – first came into use, referring to an adult Italian male who talks to his mother multiple times a day, does not do his laundry, and, of course, still lives at home with his parents. In most Western countries this would be seen as bizarre; if you found out the thirty-year-old man you were dating was still living with his mother, you might have second thoughts, right? But in Italy it is perfectly normal, and as a young Italian woman, I have encountered plenty of *mammoni*, and never once thought of judging them negatively.

There is no equivalent word when talking about girls, but I have often found myself acting as a '*mammona*' (I coined the female version of the term, since it doesn't formally exist) at various stages of my life. When I first moved out, my mother was the one I called when I didn't know how to turn on the washing machine, defrost meat, make a cake or get a tomato-sauce stain out of a new dress. My roommates thought it strange that I would call my mother instead of Googling whenever I had a question I couldn't answer, and I'd find myself desperately trying to explain that it was simply my inner *mammona* trying to make itself at home in my new apartment in London.

The concept of a *mammone* fits in perfectly with Dolce Far Niente too. It is about staying in the comfort of your home while doing (mostly) nothing.

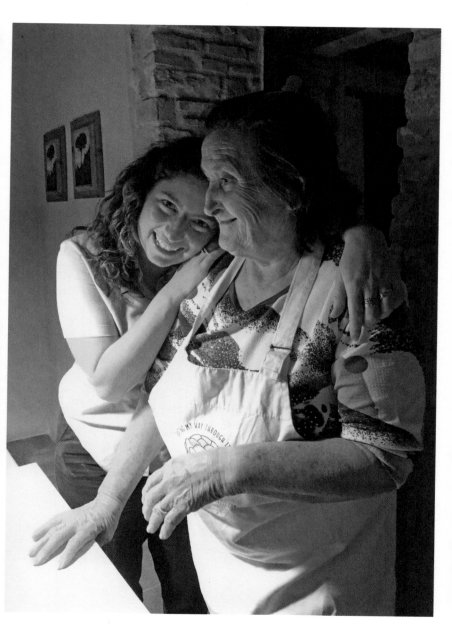

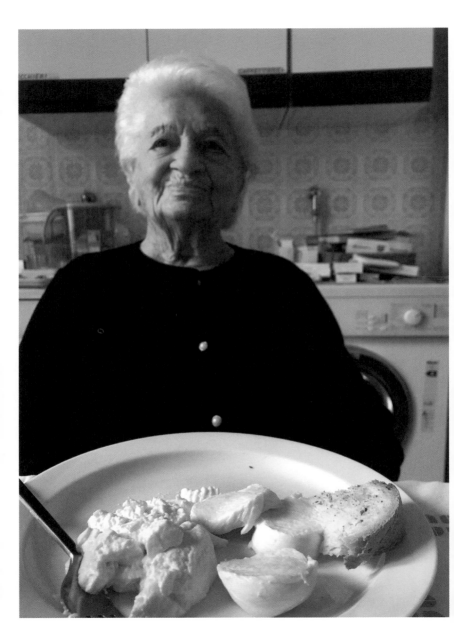

GRANDMOTHER
Nonna

The figure of the *nonna* all over Italy is elevated to mythical heights. Whenever you are hungry, you go to *nonna*. If you are sad, you go to *nonna*. If you can't sleep, you go to *nonna*. And with times changing as they are, the *nonna* is viewed as a precious cultural treasure of the past and the perfect embodiment of Italian heritage.

Since my *nonna* lives a five-hour drive away from Rome, I was only really able to see her on major holidays or long weekends while growing up. But as soon as I turned eighteen and got my driver's licence, I made sure to go and see her at least once a month, no matter how long it took to get there.

GRANDPARENTS
I nonni

Life expectancy in Italy is not only one of the highest in Europe, but in the world. As mentioned earlier, many believe the reason for Italians living so long (studies show average life expectancy is 83) is an active social life and close-knit family circle, as well as a healthy diet. It's very common for extended families to live right next to (or very close to) each other because most parents will help newlyweds with the purchase of their first home (meaning it will most likely be in the same building or right next door). This sort of family situation means that the grown children are able to work, the grandparents benefit from an active social life while taking care of the grandchildren and the grandchildren themselves are lucky enough to grow up with grandparent figures in their lives.

If you walk around any Italian city or town mid-morning, you will see a huge amount of *nonni* and *nonne* slowly strolling around with their grandchildren at the park, at the market and at the corner coffee bar. One of my favourite squares in Rome is Piazza di Testaccio. No matter what time of day, there is always some *nonni* action going on. Early in the morning, it's the women with their shopping carts, quickly making their way to the market before anyone else gets there and steals the best produce from under their noses. Mid-morning, the women disappear into their homes (cooking up something delicious) and the men slowly start strolling around the neighbourhood, finding a seat on a bench to read the newspaper, or at one of the bar's tables to play cards with their friends. At lunchtime, the square is deserted, with everyone at home, eating and then taking a nap. Then, in the afternoon – the time I like best – the kids are out of school, so the grandparents stand in groups on each corner of the square or on the benches that frame it on each side, carefully watching their grandchildren running around from one side to another.

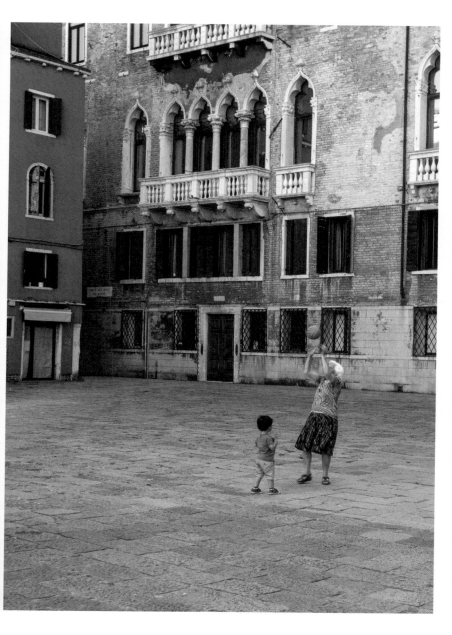

COURGETTE FRITTATA
Frittata di Zucchine

You can pretty much substitute the courgette for any vegetable you like, using the same cooking method. I've done it in the past with squash, aubergine or Swiss chard. With courgettes, I like to add fresh mint leaves once they are cooked and cooling down in a bowl, before adding the eggs. Frittata tastes even better when served at room temperature.

SERVES 4

500g courgettes
olive oil
1 garlic clove
6 eggs
salt and black pepper
grated parmigiano
   (or pecorino)

1. Wash and pat dry the courgettes. Place them on a cutting board and chop into smaller cubes.
2. In a pan, add some olive oil and a garlic clove. Once the garlic has turned golden take it out and add the courgettes.
3. Let the courgettes cook for about 10 minutes, stirring them around often. Add as much salt as you like. If they look like they are burning, you can add a little water to help them. They should not be brown and burnt. Once the courgettes are cooked, take them out of the pan and set them aside (they need to cool off a little).
4. In a bowl mix together the eggs, salt, pepper and grated cheese. Once the courgettes have cooled off a little (10 minutes is enough) add them to bowl with the egg mixture and stir.
5. Pour everything into a pan on a medium heat and let cook for about 5 minutes per side. To flip over the frittata, place a flat plate on the open side of the pan, flip onto the plate and slide it back into the pan to finish cooking the other side. After 5 minutes your frittata is ready to eat.

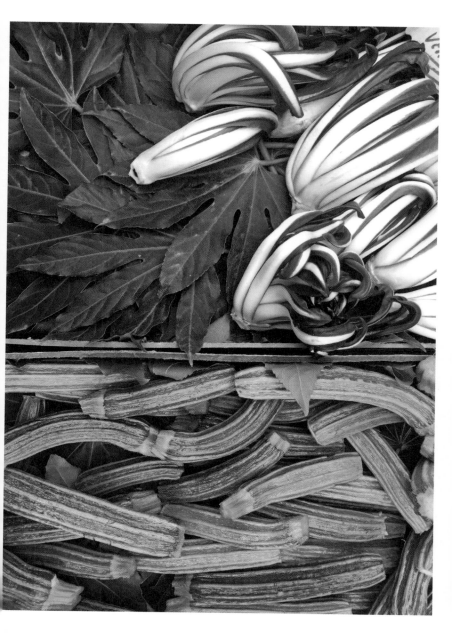

THE HOUSEDRESS
La vestaglia da casa

Something you might notice if you visit Italy (especially in smaller towns) is that all the mothers and grandmas seem to be wearing the same thing: a light blue, cotton wraparound 'dress' with some sort of decorative pattern. The housedress can also have buttons and be sleeveless, but it is almost always some shade of blue.

The housedress is partly a uniform: used for housework, it is daily wear for women in the countryside, or even the city. It is worn while performing chores like cooking or cleaning. The housedress is also very symbolic, separating domestic and social life. When an Italian woman has her housedress on that means she is 'working' and will not leave the house until she decides to take it off.

Growing up in Italy the sight of a housedress was so familiar. Nowadays, they are slowly disappearing, and only the older generations still use them on a daily basis. Whenever I see one at an open-air market, I make sure to buy it – it makes me feel nostalgic for times gone by. Plus, they are really cute! Some housedresses have been passed on from generation to generation. I recently managed to find one of my grandma's old ones. Who knows, maybe I will want to wear it when I am a *nonna* myself?

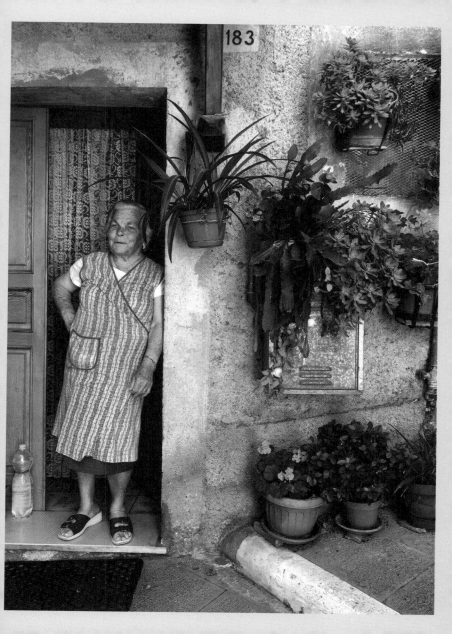

CAN I MAKE YOU A COFFEE?

Ti posso fare un caffè?

If most Italians have coffee at a bar at least once a day (see p. 39), a completely different set of social traditions governs coffee at home in the family. Whenever you enter a friend's or family member's home, you are immediately asked this question: *ti posso fare un caffè?* And even if you politely refuse the offer (perhaps you've had too much coffee that day or just don't feel like having one), the friend or family member will equally politely ignore your refusal and pull out the *moka* anyway. While it may seem like this should be in the food chapter, I felt it had to be here because just as food is a symbol of family and love in Italy, coffee is too.

Invented by a Mr Bialetti in the 1930s, the *moka* (named after the Yemeni city of Mocha) is a distinctive coffee pot which has now become a symbol of the 'made in Italy' design, synonymous with drinking coffee. Each home has at least one of these, but more often multiple ones in different sizes. And just like everything else that is food- or drink-related in Italy, people have very strong opinions on how to make the best pot of coffee. Levelled or pressed coffee powder? Hot or tepid water? Medium or low flame? So here are some simple instructions for mastering the art of using a *moka*:

1

Timing

This is a crucial part of the ritual. It takes time to make a cup of coffee: getting the pot out, measuring water and grounds, waiting for the coffee are all as important as drinking the coffee itself. It shows you care about the person, and that you are stopping whatever else you are doing to prepare them the perfect tiny cup of espresso.

2

The water

Some prefer 'clean' water, meaning bottled or filtered, while others

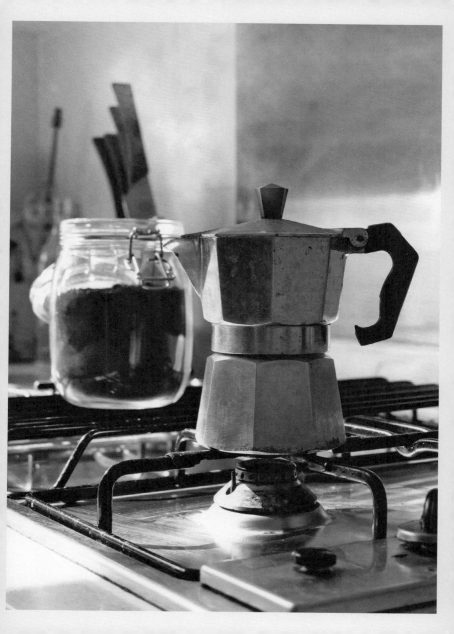

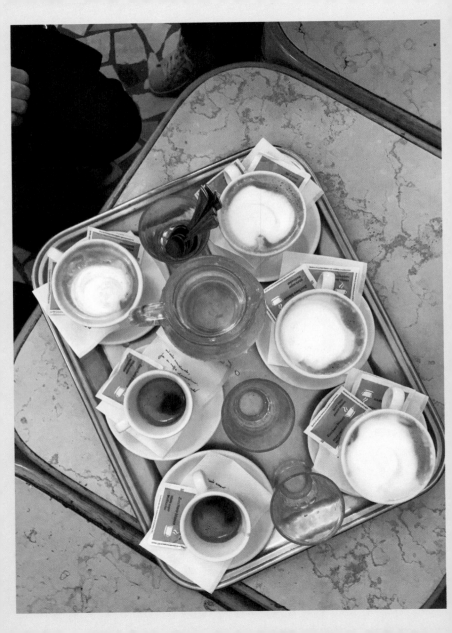

prefer tap water with all its calcium. People in Rome and Naples take great pride in their cities' tap water, giving it all (or almost all) the credit for their delicious world-famous coffee.

3
The water level

If you peek inside the water chamber of your *moka*, you will spot a little valve near the rim. There is a big discussion as to whether the valve should be covered with water or not. It's there to let the steam out, so I don't usually cover it.

4
The coffee blend

Most coffee bars will use a blend made up of 30 per cent Robusta and 70 per cent Arabica, although some prefer 100 per cent Arabica. Play around with brands and blends until you find the one that suits your personal taste.

5
The coffee powder mountain

This is probably the most controversial issue. When placing the ground coffee powder in the filter, do you create a loose little mountain or press it down? I prefer to keep it loose, but I've often pressed it down and haven't seen a huge difference.

6
The flame

The key to making the perfect-tasting espresso is keeping the flame on medium–low. If the flame is too high, the water will be pushed through the coffee very fast, losing some flavour along the way. Everything, even making the perfect coffee, needs to be done slowly in Italy.

FRIENDSHIP
L'amicizia

Very often, the closest friends become a part of the family. It always takes a little longer for Italians to trust you, but once you gain that trust and become a friend, you are a friend for life. Friendship and family in Italy are completely intertwined and totally complement each other. Oftentimes, an inner circle of friends includes a number of cousins.

CIRCLE OF FRIENDS
Comitiva

Whether you are young or old, male or female, you are always surrounded by a group of friends growing up in Italy. Usually this group, also known as your *comitiva*, will stick with you for your entire life. While I still have some very close friends from kindergarten and elementary school, my true *comitiva* was formed in high school. This means that their house was my house, my parents were their parents (and vice versa) and every single moment of free time was spent together.

If you take a walk around any Italian town right after dinnertime, you will come across countless groups of friends (of all ages) chatting until it's time to go to bed.

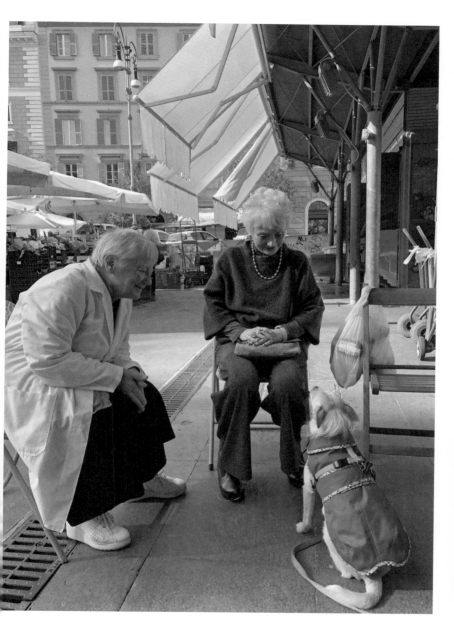

GROWING UP IN ITALY
Crescere in Italia

Whenever I lead tours through Rome, I like to chat with my clients about daily life in Italy. Somehow, what people seem to be most curious about is what it is like to grow up here, so here's a little guide:

- **From eight to thirteen years old:** at about this age Italian children get their first taste of independence. They are allowed to meet friends from the neighbourhood and wander in the streets and squares around their homes. Activities usually include *gelato*-eating, tossing a football around the piazza or park or just sitting on the steps of a fountain, chatting the afternoon away. I grew up in a neighbourhood called Rione Monti in Rome. From the outside it might seem like any other Roman neighbourhood, but as a kid it was my own little town, with its shops, cobblestoned alleys where laundry hung off the windows, school, church and ice-cream shops. After school, we were free to roam around on our own, just as long as we made it home by dinner. As kids, having this sense of independence felt amazing; we knew we had to stay within the neighbourhood (we could never cross the big roads that led to other areas), but even with this restriction we felt like adults.
- **From fourteen to eighteen years old:** the start of high school is usually the next step to social independence. Kids are allowed to drive scooters or cars with a smaller motor (50cc), and so can drive themselves to school, to friends' houses and make their way independently to any weekend activities. This is also when they are allowed to go out for a meal or two on weekends, feeling very grown up.

High school, for me, was also the time when I was finally allowed to move on from the piazza in my neighbourhood to another not too far away. And the other major change was that I was finally given permission to meet my friends after dinner. Nights were spent in Campo de Fiori, a beautiful square which my *comitiva* and which I decided to make our own for a few years. Many a weekend evening was spent just sitting around the square, chatting and chatting until it was time to go home.

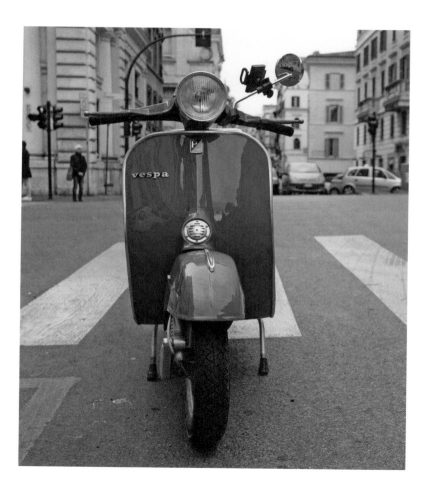

SOCIAL CLUBS
Circoli

When I was growing up, each neighbourhood used to have one or more *circoli*, and these were usually the places where the men of the neighbourhood would get together to play cards, talk about life's happenings and read the newspapers. Today, sadly, due to rising rents and changing habits, they have almost completely disappeared from the bigger cities, although happily, the situation is different in smaller towns, especially in the south. There, you will still find many of these clubs, each with a different name. Sometimes they are named after saints, meaning they are usually in charge of setting up the annual procession and fair dedicated to that saint, which each town celebrates on a different day.

These are private 'clubs', where the older retired men of the town while away their time, usually sitting on chairs right outside the entrance, people-watching. The clubs give these men a sense of identity and purpose, as well as a daily routine after they retire. Retirement in Italy is seen as positive, and there seems to be none of the fuss that goes on in Anglo-Saxon societies about how to cope with a loss of purpose. Retirement is a chance to finally relax and simply do nothing, enjoying the simple pleasures in life: Dolce Far Niente.

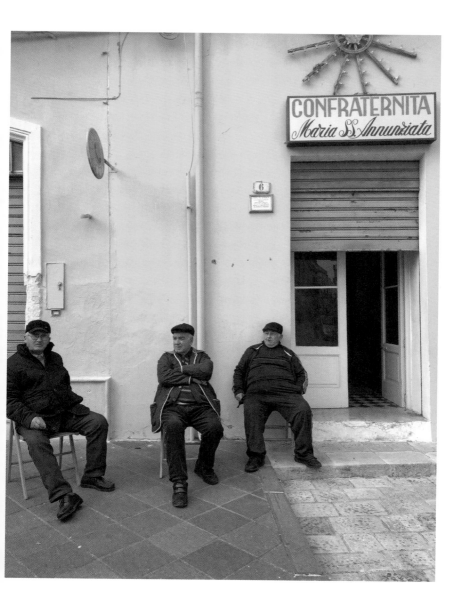

'LET'S MEET FOR A COFFEE?'

'Ci vediamo per un caffè?'

Just as I put the coffee-drinking at home section in this chapter, I decided to put this one in here too – because in Italy, asking someone to meet for a coffee simply means 'Let's meet for a chat'; it's a social situation.

While in faster-paced countries drinking coffee has become a somewhat rushed experience, whereby you dash into a shop and leave with a takeaway cup in your hand, the coffee situation in Italy is quite the opposite. I already mentioned how a pot of homemade coffee in Italy is a symbol of love, trust, family bond and so much more (see p. 14). But having said that, most of the coffee-drinking in Italy happens outside of the house, at the bar.

Even having coffee at a bar on your own is considered a social thing in Italy, since most people will go to the same bar over and over (more because of the owners and the clients than the quality of the coffee itself). Loyalty is a huge part of being Italian, so once you've picked a bar, you will keep going there for years. The owners will become your family, and you'll end up seeing the same faces, day after day. And if they caught you going to another bar in the same neighbourhood? It would be as if you had cheated on them. It's a very big no-no.

I used to frequent the same bar for years and years, taking it for granted, until one morning, about five years ago, I walked in for my usual order and the owners shared the horrible news that they would be closing at the end of the week. My heart shattered. It felt like I had lost somebody from my family, a fixture in my everyday life.

Quite simply, some of the best memories of life in Italy are built around standing at the bar, sipping on piping-hot espresso.

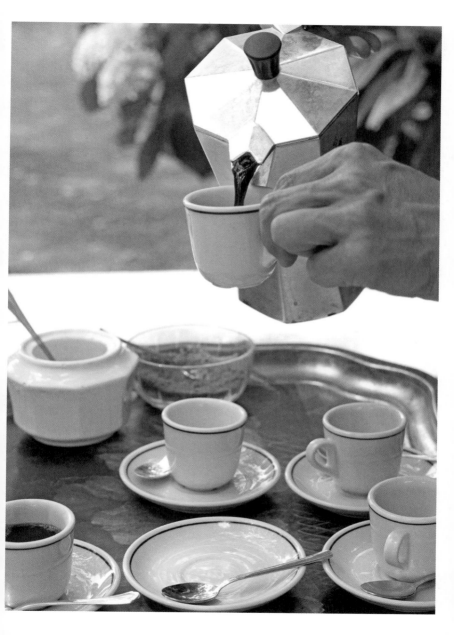

RULES FOR THE COFFEE BAR

BEING IN A NEW COUNTRY CAN BE OVERWHELMING, SO HERE ARE A FEW RULES FOR YOU TO FOLLOW WHEN ORDERING COFFEE IN ITALY. (YES, WE REALLY DO HAVE VERY STRICT COFFEE RULES!)

1. When ordering an espresso, *never* call it an espresso. If you simply say *'un caffè per favore'* ('a coffee, please') you will be served a little ceramic cup of coffee. An espresso in Italy *is* a *caffè*.

2. No milk after 11 pm (so this means no cappuccinos). Italians believe a hot cup of milk too late in the day will mess with your digestion, so if you really feel you need milk, order a *caffè macchiato* instead, and you will be served a coffee with just a little bit of milk.

3. You will never see an Italian order a *caffè doppio* (double shot), so if you feel like you really need to have two coffees' worth, just make a second trip to the bar; you won't be the only one!

4. Try drinking your *caffè 'al banco'*, which means sipping it standing up at the bar. This is a good way to chat with locals, people-watch and get to know the owner and barista. If you keep up this routine, you won't even have to ask for your order after a while, as they will remember it and serve it with a smile.

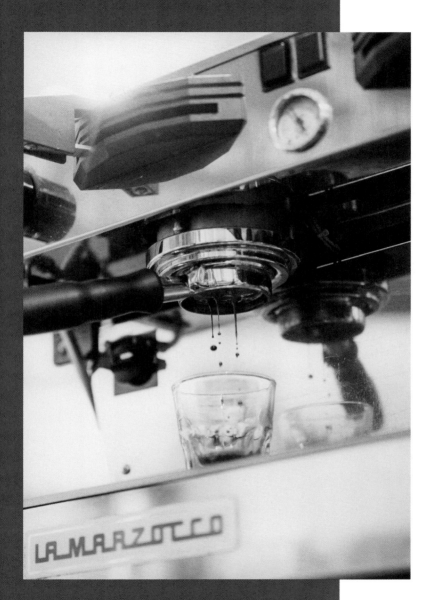

THE SQUARE
La piazza

Each neighbourhood or small town has a main piazza. This is where people get most of their shopping done, and it serves as a sort of open-air theatre for those who pass by. Pretty much every square in Italy has the same features: a post office for getting mail sorted and bills paid, an *alimentari* to buy pantry goods and fresh milk, a *fruttivendolo* to get fresh fruit and vegetables, a bank to get cash and a bar for satisfying cravings (whatever they may be) at any time of the day.

The most sacred parts of any piazza are the benches, placed either at the centre or on either side of the square. This is where the older inhabitants of the town sit to observe what's going on in town. They are front-row seats to the best show in town: life. Wedding proposals, birthday invitations, quarrels and rumours all go through the main square.

Observing any Italian piazza, it may seem as though the people there are doing nothing, but they are actually making sure everything runs smoothly, finding comfort in following the same routine every day for years. People-watching (or 'life-watching', as I like to call it) is a perfect example of Dolce Far Niente.

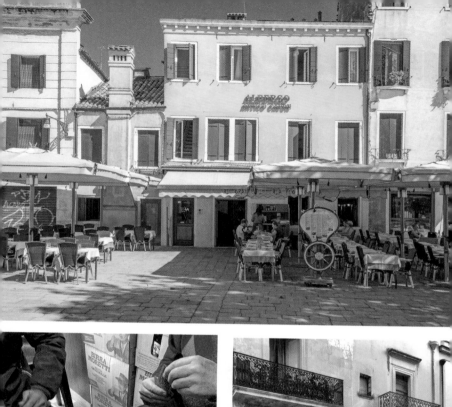

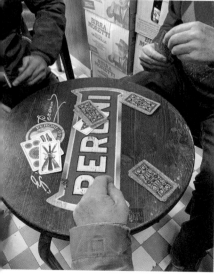

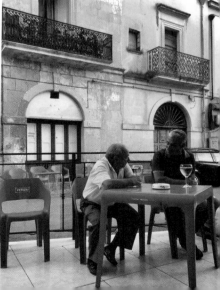

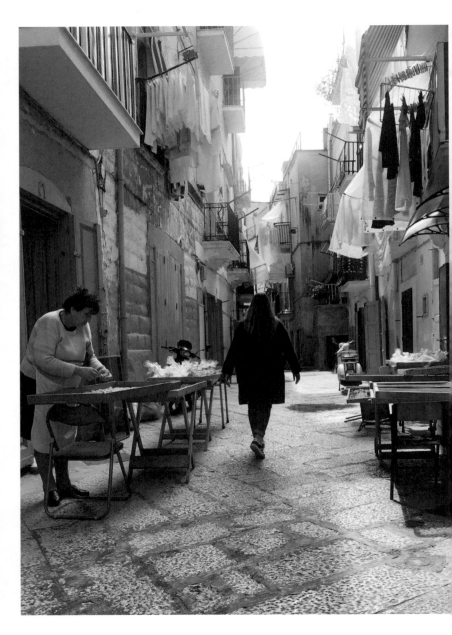

TAKING A WALK
Passeggiata

This is probably one of my favourite Italian rituals, but *passeggiata* is no simple walk: it takes place every evening between 5 and 8 pm, when the light is golden and work is over. On weekdays, it is a chance to socialise after work and before dinner. On weekends, the whole family will take part, especially on Sunday evenings, when people need to walk off all the food from lunch.

In any big city or small town, you will see people slowly strolling up and down pedestrian streets all over the historic centre, or along the boardwalk if it's by the sea. People of all ages take part in the *passeggiata*: you might see couples pushing strollers, teenagers planning something mischievous while away from their parents, mothers sitting (or standing) at a bar sipping on coffee, grandparents sitting on benches and kids chasing after a football or eating *gelato*.

This is the time of day to relax and do whatever you prefer, but it is also a time to show off – a new pair of shoes or new jacket, perhaps – and people will be strutting about, turning the pavement into a catwalk.

The *passeggiata* is not to be confused with walking for exercise. Although you might get some steps in, the point of this walk is to take it slowly and stop as often as possible.

PERSONAL SPACE

By definition, personal space is 'the cylinder of air surrounding each person, which people consider to be an extension of their body'. Italians have no idea what this is. And while some people might find it frustrating, it's one of the things I love most about Italy.

There are different theories as to why Italians have no sense of personal space, but it's most likely because Italy is an expressive country, traditionally devoted to living a communal life, centred around piazzas and churches. It could also be a throwback to times of scarcity, when people had to rely on each other to survive, making them emotionally and physically closer.

Italians' naturally outgoing personalities encourage the expression of emotions, whether it is crying, screaming or kissing. It's common to see couples embracing in public, neighbours in the midst of screaming fights and friends walking down the street, arm in arm. In conversation, Italians (both men and women) tend to stand very close together, often touching one another's arms or shoulders.

Perhaps as an extension of this, in families, there are no secrets whatsoever and nothing is off-limits. So during big family reunions, it's normal for the various grandmas, aunts and uncles to greet you with, 'Have you been eating a little too much pasta? You seem ... rounder', and follow up with a squeeze on the cheek or a pat on the belly. I found this very challenging during my teen years, but as an adult I've learned to embrace it, accepting it in the spirit in which it is intended – namely, their way of showing affection. So much so, that when I moved to London, I deeply missed my grandma telling me I was chubby, my local barista grabbing my hand before giving me my coffee, the woman selling flowers on the corner asking me a thousand questions on my love life ...

Here are some other typically Italian space-invading habits:

Double kiss
In Italy, you only shake someone's hand on the first encounter. Thereafter, you greet them with a double peck on the cheeks (one for each side). This is true not only for family and friends, but also in business and work situations.

Queuing
There is no such thing as standing in an orderly queue for Italians. Don't be offended if the person behind you is so close that their elbow touches yours. They just can't help themselves.

Conversation
No matter who you are talking to in Italy, chances are they will stand very close to you, look directly into your eyes and touch your arm when they want you to pay close attention to something important. It might seem scary at first, but I think it's just their way of showing that you are being included in their conversation and they really care about you. With the rise of text messages, this can be a sweet reminder that we should all try to communicate in a more 'human' way every now and then.

HOW CAN I INCORPORATE SOME OF THESE CONCEPTS INTO MY LIFE?

Dolce Far Niente is a way of life, and here in Italy it's built into every little thing we do. Don't feel you have to try to recreate exactly the various concepts I explain in this chapter, but use them as inspiration, introducing them into your life in whichever way possible. This has to be done slowly, of course, in typical Dolce Far Niente style. Take your time trying out a few of these things and, I can assure you, you will find joy and happiness in doing them.

1
Take time to enjoy your coffee

Create your own coffee routine at your local coffee shop, even if it's just once a week. If there isn't one where you can sip your coffee while standing at the bar and chatting with the people around you, try sitting and people-watching for as long as you can spare. Try not looking at your phone or a book, just let your mind wander aimlessly as you watch life go by. The ultimate in Dolce Far Niente.

2
Spend time with someone much older than you

Growing up in Italy taught me to always respect my elders, regardless of whether or not they're related to me. I find great peace in listening to stories from someone older than me – it allows me to dream and takes my mind off things. If you see an older person sitting alone on a bench, stop and have a chat with them. They will most likely be more than happy to tell you a story that will make your day brighter and help you put things in perspective.

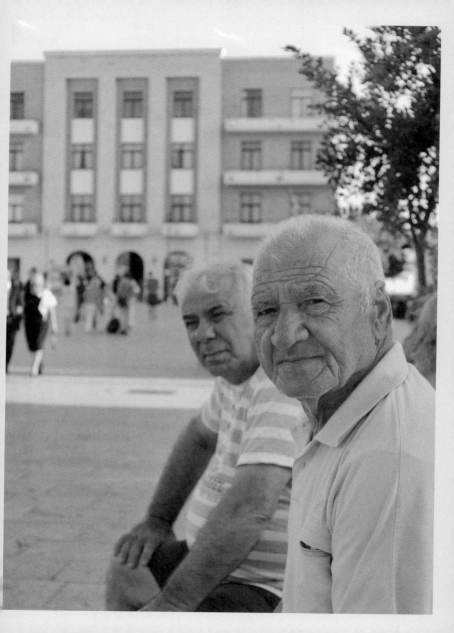

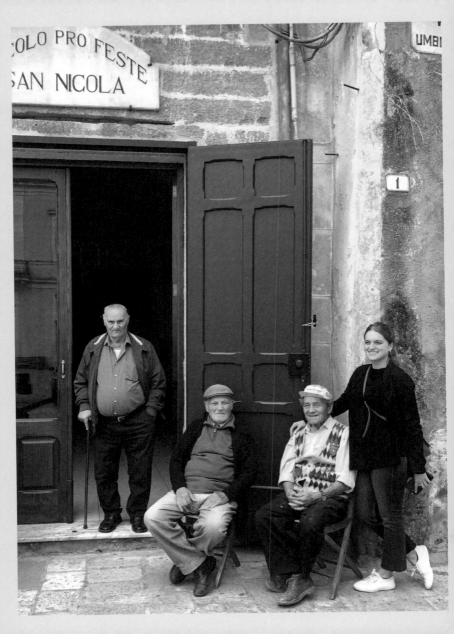

3

Take a walk every day

We all know that walking is beneficial to your physical health, but Italians use it as a way to keep themselves sane mentally too. Whether you are alone or with friends, try to take a walk before or after work. If you can't fit one in at either of those times, how about not eating lunch at your desk, and taking a walk then instead? It will clear your mind and you will feel refreshed and revitalised back at your desk. And keep in mind that for these purposes, it's not the quantity of your walk (steps), but the quality. In other words: you should stop to smell the roses – literally – or stroke a puppy or talk to the postman.

Be more passionate. Italians put passion and love into almost everything they do. Think about one or two things you enjoy in life, and make sure to do them once a week, every week.

4

Value your friendships

A close circle of friends is so important. However, maintaining friendships is not always easy and takes a lot of effort on both sides. With the rise of technology and social media, we have become too reliant on online interactions, which are replacing the real and more 'human' ones. Try reconnecting with some friends and make the effort to meet up with somebody you haven't seen in a while. Or create a weekly (or monthly) tradition with a closer friend who you don't see as much as you used to. You might have to make some changes in your schedule to accommodate this, but it will be so worth it.

5

Start up your own *circoli*

There may not be a social club you can hang out in locally, but that doesn't mean you can't start your own version of one – a book club, a dining or cookery club or some other sort of activity once a month is a good way to create a space outside of your home where you and a group of friends can get together. What you do there is not the important part – the point is to be with people and take the time to socialise with no real goal.

6

Dress for your chores

Ok, I'm not suggesting you go straight out and buy a housedress (but by all means, please do, if that appeals). But you can get into the spirit by wearing something that's just for when you are doing chores at home. It can be a designated apron, a comfy sweatshirt or anything else that makes taking care of your own space feel special and gives you pride in the seemingly smallest of tasks.

While both family and friends are a fundamental part of the Italian lifestyle, I am also aware that not everyone has a huge family waiting for them at home or a tight-knit circle of friends to meet up with for a coffee or drink every afternoon. Each person has a different living and social situation, but these concepts can be easily adapted to all. Dolce Far Niente is more about yourself and the way you feel, so while the people around you are important, it doesn't entirely depend on them.

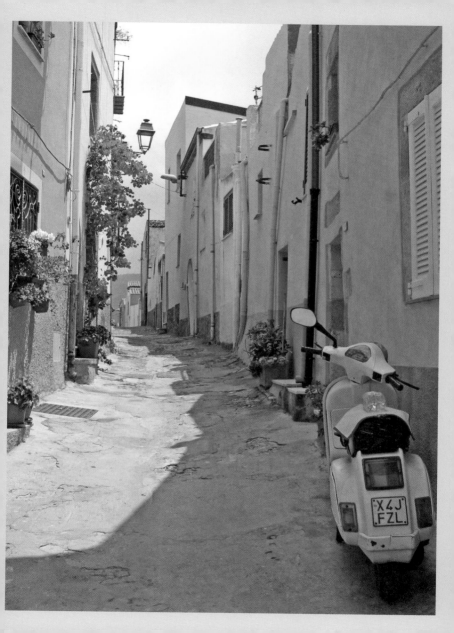

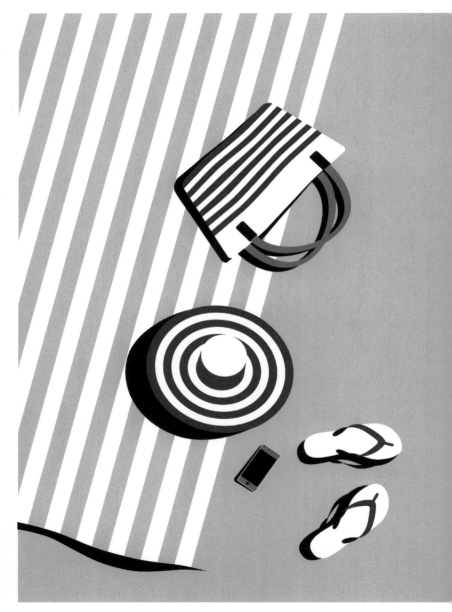

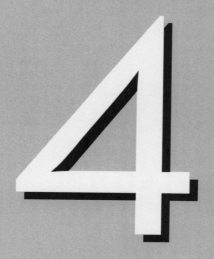

LEISURE

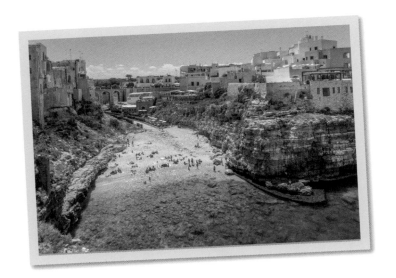

LEISURE
Tempo libero

If there is one thing Italians know how to do extremely well, it's cutting a razor-sharp line between work and leisure. If they feel they need a break from work, they will take one.

By law, Italians have a minimum of four holiday weeks per year, and if you happen to work for yourself, you can shut down your shop, restaurant or office whenever you please and for however long you want. On top of that, there are ten national holidays and endless smaller ones which differ for each city or town.

Big cities like Rome, Florence or Milan are like ghost towns during the month of August. People shut down their businesses for three weeks and head to the beach or the countryside, where they completely shut off their brains until they return to work in September for a fresh start.

During the rest of the year, most people's free time is spent with friends or family, meeting for coffee, taking a walk, watching a movie or playing a game of cards. Socialising is probably Italians' favourite activity (after eating!); just sitting around, chatting about life with friends, can feel like pure bliss compared to the stress that so often comes with work.

Think about what makes you happy; in a situation of stress and anxiety what brings you peace? Of course, the answer is different for each person, and there is no right or wrong way of doing it. Dolce Far Niente is a way of life, but it's very personal too. Learning to make time for yourself and doing the things *you* enjoy helps you to make better decisions, to focus on the good things and to gain perspective and insight in your life. Think of it as your very own personal version of self-care. However, I believe that in today's world, we are expected to practise 'self-care' not for our own benefit, but in order to recharge, so that we can be a more productive individual the following day. Importantly, while Dolce Far Niente can be seen as a temporary version of self-care, it is actually a lifestyle that should slowly become a part of your daily, weekly, yearly routine.

In this chapter I talk about a few of the things that bring happiness and calm into Italians' everyday life. Hopefully they will inspire you to slow down a little – because Dolce Far Niente is all about taking things slowly. Very slowly.

THE BEACH
La spiaggia

What Italians look forward to all year, perhaps more than anything else, is the beach. Going to the beach for an Italian is not only about the scenery, but also the routine that surrounds it: the Italian beach experience.

A beach in Italy at the peak of summer is perfect for observing just how the Italians relax and embrace the art of Dolce Far Niente. Yes, there is chaos everywhere, but it is a gratifying chaos. An Italian beach is not only beautiful water and sand, it's a gym, a catwalk, a restaurant, a market, a beauty salon and a reading room.

A lot of Italians opt to go to a *stabilimento*: a privately owned beach club where you can pay for a sunbed and an umbrella for the whole day. There will also be a bar/restaurant, as well as showers. The first thing you'd notice when you go to one of these is that people aren't scattered all over the place haphazardly. Instead, there are endless rows of perfectly ordered umbrellas and sunbeds.

As with most other things, when it comes to the beach, Italians are creatures of habit and tend to go to the same one for most of their lives. At certain beach clubs, families can even rent their spot for the entire summer season, ensuring that they get the exact same spot from year to year. But this can get expensive, and many people prefer to go next door to the *spiaggia libera*. There are no clubs, it is publicly owned and free of charge, so you just lay your towel on the sand wherever you please.

I like both types of beach and switch around from day to day. When you have children though, the *stabilimento* is the way to go, if you can afford it, because of all the associated comforts.

Since August is when most people are on holiday, that is when beaches all over Italy get crowded. And I mean *really* crowded. So if you choose the free beach, you have to prepare: getting there early in the morning (around 9 am) is a must, and since you will most likely be spending the whole day

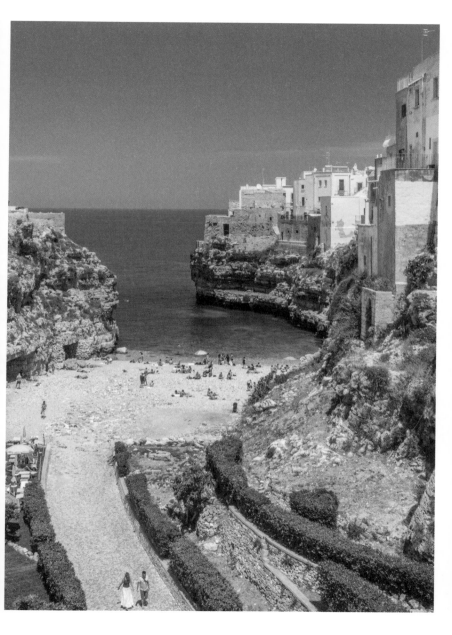

there, you should take a packed lunch, water and snacks. Be prepared to have no personal space whatsoever – you will basically be sitting underneath the same umbrella as the family next to you. But on the positive side, by the end of the day you will have become part of that Italian family!

Beach routine

Italians have a strict routine when it comes to their children and the beach. They bring them early in the morning, when the sun is – according to Italian doctors – at its healthiest (it's strongest between 12 and 3 pm, meaning it can be harmful to the skin), and will let them go in the sea later, when the coolness of the water is a relief. When the kids come out of the water, they are immediately changed into a second bathing costume, giving the first one a chance to dry. Doctors in Italy actually recommend beach time for kids, insisting that the iodine in the air is beneficial to their lungs. This means some people will try to get their kids out to the beach for the whole three-month summer break.

For at least two hours after eating, children are not allowed to go in the water, for fear of messing with their digestion (see p. 78). This can only mean one thing: naptime. Right after lunch, you will suddenly notice the beach quietens down, and most mothers and children will be lying next to each other, fast asleep. The *nonni* and *nonne* will also be sleeping on the sunbeds next door, while the young adults will most likely be working on their suntans.

One of the things Italians love about spending time at the beach is the routine. As with everything else, they love the familiar, and tend to do the same thing each and every summer. This is something I came to notice once I was older, and today, as an adult, I find it extremely comforting. People like to book the same spot every year, which means they get to know their neighbours and form a tight bond with them. The mums become good friends, the grandparents walk slowly up and down the beach together and the kids will

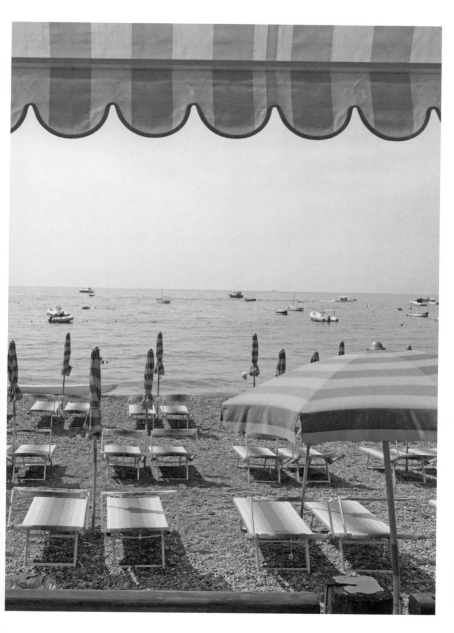

play and share their toys all summer long. In fact, most Italians have 'summer friends' whom they only see for two or three months a year, for years and years.

Lunch at the beach

Lunch, as ever, is sacred, and while on the beach, for most Italians, it will be something light – like a cold pasta salad or a sandwich overflowing with mozzarella and tomatoes – in southern Italy things are quite different. After years and years of summer holidays in the very southern tip of the boot, I have observed and come to love how people eat lunch at the beach there. It's a very serious affair.

Coolers are filled with trays of lasagna, aubergine parmigiana or *pasta al forno* – things that can easily be shared in generous portions and feed a family – with a whole watermelon for dessert and peaches and cookies for snacks. The idea is that there is enough food for your whole family, your friends and any extra people who seem hungry.

I tend to cook up something a little lighter, usually some variation of a rice or pasta salad. Lately, I've been substituting the rice for farro, because I love its texture and rich, nutty flavour. And through my many years of Italian beach training, I've learned always to bring a lot more than I think I'll need, since there is always someone who's forgotten to bring their own lunch.

SUMMER FARRO SALAD
Insalata estiva di farro

You can boil the farro the night before going to the beach and add the rest of the ingredients the next morning. For the cheese, I use *ricotta salata* or *cacioricotta*, which I know can be difficult to find abroad. It's a mix between an aged cheese and ricotta with a very salty and tangy flavour. It can easily be substituted by feta.

SERVES 4

300g farro
1 red onion
2 tbsp white
 wine vinegar
200g cherry tomatoes
1 cucumber
1 carrot
olive oil
salt
handful of capers
100g ricotta salata
 (or feta)
generous bunch
 of rocket or leaves
 of your choice

1. Bring a pot of salted water to the boil and then add the farro. Once it is cooked (usually about 15 minutes), drain and run under cold water to stop the cooking process and cool the farro down. Transfer to a bowl and set aside.
2. Chop the red onion and put in a bowl with the white wine vinegar. Leave to marinate (about 15 minutes), stirring every now and then.
3. Dice the tomatoes, cucumber and carrot and put in another bowl. Add the olive oil and salt and stir.
4. Add the cooled farro to the vegetables and add more olive oil and salt if needed.
5. Just before serving, add the capers, crumbled cheese, rocket and the marinated onions. Mix together, place in a Tupperware and head to the beach!

THE TOP FIVE BEACHES IN ITALY

TO GET A REAL FEEL OF AN ITALIAN SUMMER, TRY VISITING ONE OR MORE OF THESE BEACHES ON YOUR NEXT TRIP TO ITALY:

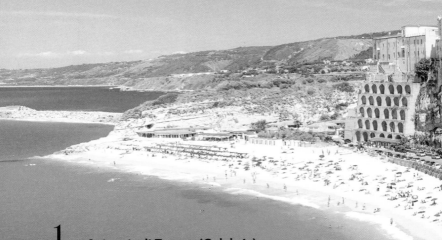

1. **Spiaggia di Tropea (Calabria)**

2. **Torre dell'Orso (Puglia)**

3. **Punta Prosciutto (Puglia)**

4. **Cala Mariolu (Sardegna)**

5. **San Vito lo Capo (Sicilia)**

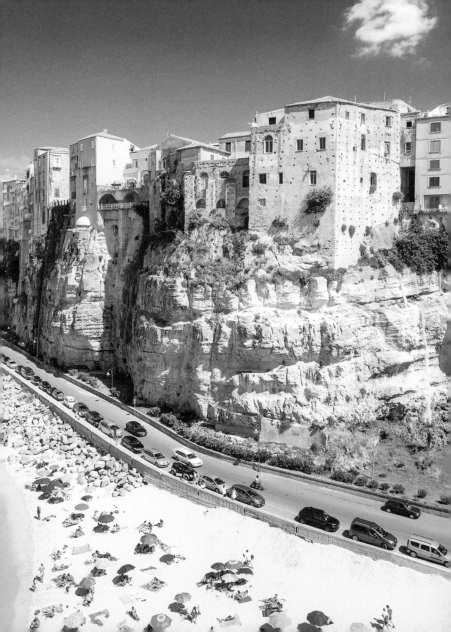

CLOSING HOURS
Orario di chiusura

If you've ever been to Italy, you might have noticed that in the smaller towns most shops close between 1.30 and 4.30 pm. This is because people go home for lunch and a nap before returning to the workplace in the afternoon, a tradition which has slowly disappeared in the bigger cities.

While it may seem strange that people can just shut up shop for a few hours and go home to eat and rest, the reason why they are able to do so is because so many still have small family-run businesses in little towns all over Italy, especially in the south. But as I said earlier, even in bigger cities where small shops are slowly disappearing and being substituted by offices, eating a sandwich in front of your computer screen is unthinkable.

With post offices, banks and shops closing at lunchtime in some places, it can make it near impossible to get anything done during a break. But if we stop to think about it, do we actually need to do or buy a particular thing right then and there? Probably not. So instead of getting frustrated, I take it as a cue to use my break for actual relaxing and embracing the art of Dolce Far Niente – because there really is nothing else I can do.

What's more, in the summertime, the only refuge for Italians during the hottest hours of the day, when temperatures can easily reach 40 °C, is their family home. So if you find yourself travelling to Italy in the summer, try to adopt the naptime tradition – you'll be glad you did.

A LITTLE FUN IN THE WORKPLACE

A few months ago, I took a lovely American family on an afternoon food tour through Rome. We arrived at one of the stops, sat down at a table and placed our order. After a couple of minutes, the owner of the restaurant started singing out of his karaoke machine without a care in the world, as if he was at home, in his own living room. At first, I was concerned that my clients would be annoyed by the loud singing, but I explained that sometimes Italians just do as they want, irrespective of where they are and who they are with, and we all laughed and listened happily. This is just one example of how Italians manage to keep things on the 'lighter' side. Sure, they're at work and maybe not really in the mood to be there, so why not sing a song to make it better?

Of course, most of us can't just pull out a karaoke machine in the middle of the workplace and start singing, but if you feel you need a break, why not take one? That's Dolce Far Niente!

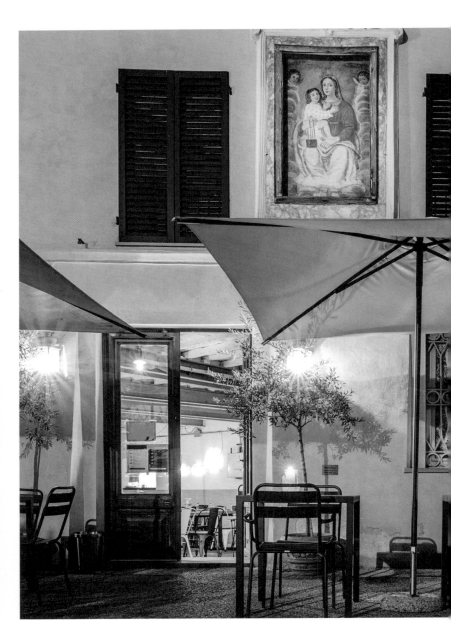

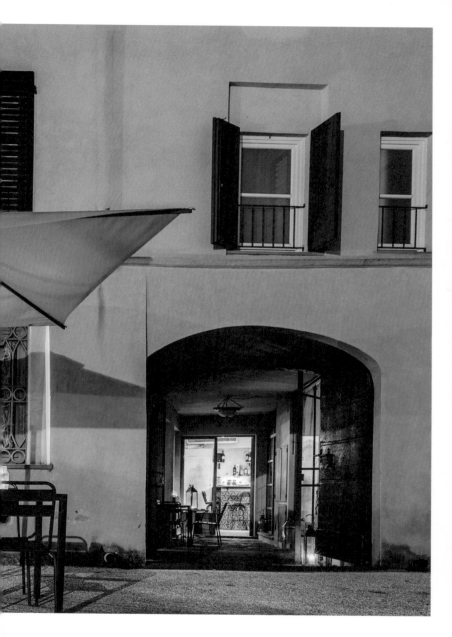

GOOD IMPRESSIONS
Bella figura

'*Bella figura*' literally translates as 'beautiful figure' but is used to mean 'good impression'. This is integral to Italian culture, being instilled in children from a very young age and sticking with them through adulthood.

Children go to school wearing clean and neatly put-together outfits (uniforms are very rare, only in certain private Catholic schools), and the same goes for adults, whether it's for their afternoon *passeggiata* through town (see p. 131) or for meetings at work. But it doesn't stop at clothing. It's also about the way you act in public and making the best possible impression in all areas of life. What else could we expect from a country that has been creating beauty for centuries? Beauty is everywhere in Italy, from that perfect plate of pasta to a exquisitely tailored suit. Italians strongly believe that being surrounded by beauty is beneficial to a happier life.

Bella figura is evident in all areas of Italian life: a beautifully laid table for guests, a perfectly cared-for flower garden, an immaculately cleaned house, a teenager wearing the latest trendy sneakers. It even extends to the Italian who would rather miss the bus and be late for an engagement than arrive on time all frazzled and sweaty. Better late and in order than on time and a mess.

Italians are known to be some of the most generous and hospitable people on earth, and this stems not only from wanting guests to feel welcome, but also from a wish to make a positive impression. That is why if you are ever invited for a meal at an Italian home, the table will be filled with enough food to feed an army, so as not to make the hosts look cheap. I can't tell you how many times I have left a meal at someone's home in Italy feeling completely stuffed (in a good way) – and with gifts to bring back to my parents (usually food).

For those who did not grow up with it, *bella figura* might seem strange or excessive, but for Italians, looking – and therefore feeling – good is a fundamental part of their existence and of what it means to be Italian. And while it might seem a little superficial to an outsider, *bella figura* means being able to own your actions, behaving with respect, being comfortable in your own skin, appreciating good design, being hospitable and combining beauty with necessity in the most harmonious way possible. It also means appreciating these qualities in others and noticing beauty everywhere you go. So from this perspective, the fancy shoes and perfectly tailored suit are just extras; the important lesson is that life is already very beautiful, but we can always add that little extra touch of personalised beauty, in whatever way we choose to interpret it.

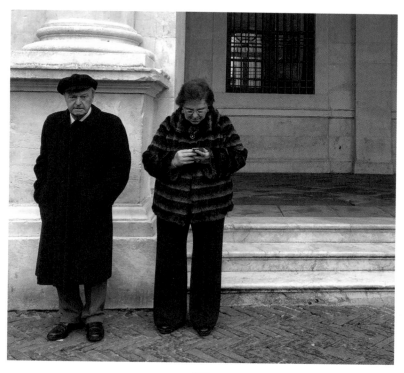

'SORRY FOR THE DELAY':
BEING LATE (THE ITALIAN WAY)
'Scusa il ritardo!'

Despite a reputation for being late, Italians are always punctual for anything work-related. But it is the case that they have a different concept of time when it comes to more personal engagements. I think this comes from the fact that Italians don't like to feel rushed or constrained by a specific time slot. If you try to get an appointment with an electrician, for example, or arrange a delivery to your home in Italy, they will most likely not give you an exact time; instead, they'll say something like, 'I'll be there before lunch'.

When talking about Italians and punctuality, there are two people in my life that come to mind: my father and my best friend, Emanuele.

My father wouldn't dream of being late for a work meeting, but whenever the time came for us to all go to a dinner party at someone's house, something strange would happen to his timekeeping. If we were invited for 8.30 pm, my mother, sister and I would want to set out at 8.15 pm, but my father would not leave the house before 8.28 pm. After years of this happening, over and over, we still haven't managed to figure out why he refuses to get to a dinner party on time. But then again, on the very few occasions we did manage to arrive punctually, we were the only ones to do so. Maybe my dad was right, after all?

As for Emanuele, he has been my best friend for over twenty years, and while I love him very much, his tardiness drives me insane. I'm sure this is something that is common to many nationalities, but I've always thought of it as one of his most Italian traits. In any case, I just know that no matter what time we arrange to meet, he will show up at least twenty minutes late.

When you challenge someone in Italy as to why they are late, they will tell you, 'I just had to have coffee at the bar before meeting you', or, 'My mum called to ask what I want to eat tonight'. And excuses like these can get you out of any situation in Italy, no matter how late you are.

So after years of feeling completely frustrated by all the tardiness that surrounded me (having been known as that person who is always early or perfectly on time), I decided it was time to ignore the American side of my brain, and accept this for what it is. Quite simply, people in Italy are relaxed; there is never a feeling of being in a rush, and if someone is late, it is probably because of something that has brought joy to their life – like that coffee or that phone call from their mother.

This is Dolce Far Niente in action: letting go of the pressure and anxiety society puts on us about time management. Sure, being on time to work is important, but do we really need to feel like we are constantly in a rush? Studies show that individuals who live life in a time-urgent way tend to engage in self-defeating behaviours such as excessive worry with regard to schedules and deadlines and doing several activities at the same time, while not really taking the time to enjoy any of them.

SPEAKING DIALECT
Dialetto

The distinction between work and free time is so great that Italians even speak differently in both situations. 'Proper' Italian is taught in schools and used on TV; but Italians also all speak their own dialect, specific to the region they are from. Some dialects are stronger than others: some don't even sound like Italian, while others just have a very strong and distinctive accent. Up until the unification of Italy, most people only spoke their own dialect. Italian is said to have originated from Tuscany, where the 'perfect' language was spoken by those of a higher class. Slowly, people from all over Italy started mixing some of their dialect words with the official language, creating what we know today as 'Italian'. However, most Italians are perfectly bilingual, speaking both the official language and their own local dialect. In fact, wherever you find yourself in Italy, you will notice that the majority of people speak proper Italian in more formal situations (if you speak some Italian you will be able to understand them), but in the comfort of their homes or just hanging out with friends, they will quickly switch to their own local dialect (even if you speak some Italian you won't be able to understand a word).

I remember first becoming aware of another dialect when spending a summer in the deep south, in the part of Puglia known as Salento. Day after day, I heard the word 'crai' in all sorts of contexts. To me, Crai was the name of a popular supermarket chain down south, but when I finally plucked up courage to ask one of my friends why everyone seemed to be so obsessed with it she looked at me with a puzzled expression, laughed hysterically and then explained: 'The word crai means tomorrow!' In 'proper' Italian tomorrow is domani, but the word has always brought a smile to my face ever since that time.

So in case you find yourself travelling to Italy and wanting to blend in, here are a few common words in dialect (the locals will be very impressed!):

Beddha mia (BELLA MIA)	Salento (very southern tip of Puglia, around Lecce	Literally 'My beautiful girl'; an enthusiastic way of saying hi to a girl (or when you just can't remember her name!)
Ajò (DAI ANDIAMO)	Sardegna	'Come on, let's go' (when you want somebody to get moving)
Ganzo! (BELLO)	Tuscany	Expression of unconditional admiration towards people or situations
Daje! (FORZA, DAI!)	Rome	Used as an encouragement, but can also mean 'Yes, ok'
Cumpà (EHI AMICO MIO)	Sicily	'Hey, my friend!'
Uhè Uhè (Ciao)	Naples and Amalfi coast area	An informal salutation

PRE-DINNER DRINKS
Aperitivo

One of the most popular 'activities' for Italians is meeting up after work for an *aperitivo* – otherwise known as a pre-dinner drink.

Between 6.30 and 8 pm, groups of friends and work colleagues all over Italy will meet up for what is usually a bitter cocktail or wine-based drink, along with some light snacks. The reason why the most popular pre-dinner drinks are bitter in taste is because they are said to stimulate hunger, preparing the stomach for food.

Here are a few of the most popular drinks for *aperitivo*:

APEROL SPRITZ

If you take a walk around any town in Italy in the late afternoon, you will see people sipping on this bright orange drink. Originating in the Venice area, it has now become a staple across the country.

SERVES 1

75ml Prosecco
50ml Aperol
25ml soda water (a dash)

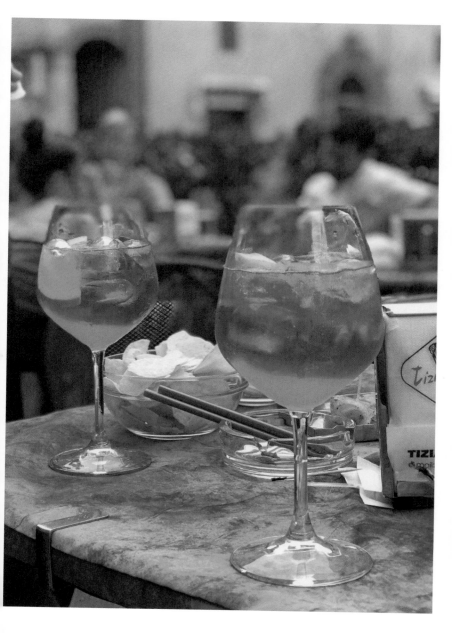

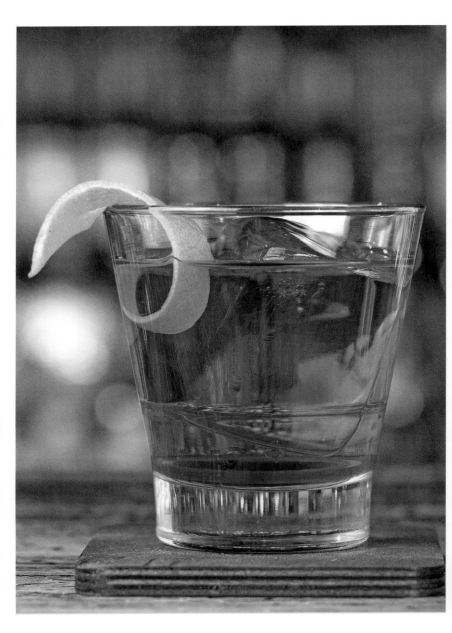

CAMPARI SODA

One of the least alcoholic drinks, this is served in Italy in a distinctive bottle, pre-mixed (it was the first drink to be sold this way). It's a mixture of Campari and soda water, so you can easily make your own at home. Fill a highball glass with ice. Pour in the Campari first, then the soda and stir gently.

SERVES 1

60ml Campari
soda water (enough to fill the rest of the glass)
orange slice

NEGRONI

Similar to an Americano in taste, this is one of the strongest *aperitivo* drinks because of the gin. Recognisable by its dark orange colour and bitter flavour, it's easy to make at home.

SERVES 1

25ml gin
25ml vermouth rosso
25ml Campari

Traditionally, whenever you order one of these drinks at a bar in Italy, you will also be served a few simple nibbles: olives, crisps and nuts.

It is also acceptable to have a light *aperitivo* before lunch, usually a Campari soda or a glass of Prosecco. I've seen this a lot in smaller towns in the south of Italy, where people close up their shops at midday, go to the bar for an *aperitivo* and then make their way home for lunch.

MUSIC
Musica

Music is everywhere in Italy. From when you are a baby to a teenager and then an adult, it is constantly playing from people's homes, cars and shops. Nowadays, people listen to all genres, but what really makes this country unique is the folk music, also known as *'musica popolare'*. Because national unification came so late, most regions in Italy still retain a specific kind of musical tradition that reflects their culture and history.

I grew up in a big city, so listening to live performances of traditional Roman folk music was difficult, and to do so I had to go to smaller towns outside of the city, in the area known as *'i castelli'*. Big cities all over Italy have struggled to keep traditions like music and dance alive, but luckily, small towns continue to do so.

When I started spending my summers in southern Italy, specifically in Salento, a whole new world of folk music opened up to me. In this area, music is an integral part of everyday life. All year long, and especially in the summer months, towns organise fairs where you will see people playing their traditional music, known as *'pizzica'*. During these gatherings, people of all ages (and I mean *all* ages, from infants to grandparents) embrace the beauty of life through music, singing and dancing like there is no tomorrow.

When I first found myself at one of these *pizzica* evenings, I was confused as to why so many people were dancing and singing until late at night: didn't they have to get up early for work? Weren't the kids tired and ready for bed? But I soon realised that yes, people did have to get up for work and school the next day – but who cares? Life is short, and people in these small towns truly embrace the important things, dancing the night away with friends and family without a care in the world. They can worry about their problems tomorrow, today is all about living in the moment. This is exactly where Dolce Far Niente is so fundamental to a careless yet happy lifestyle: live in the present, enjoy every single moment as if it were the last.

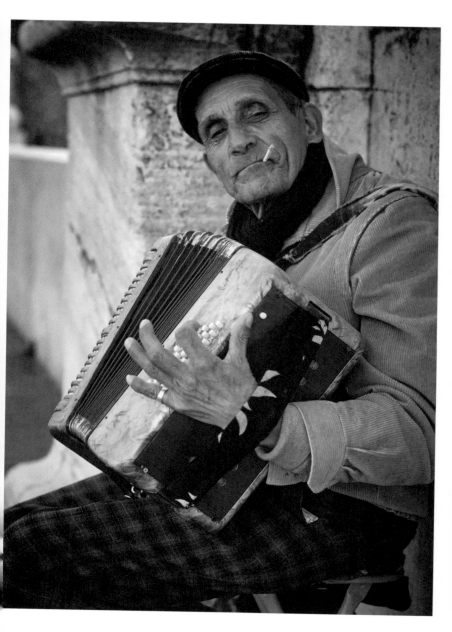

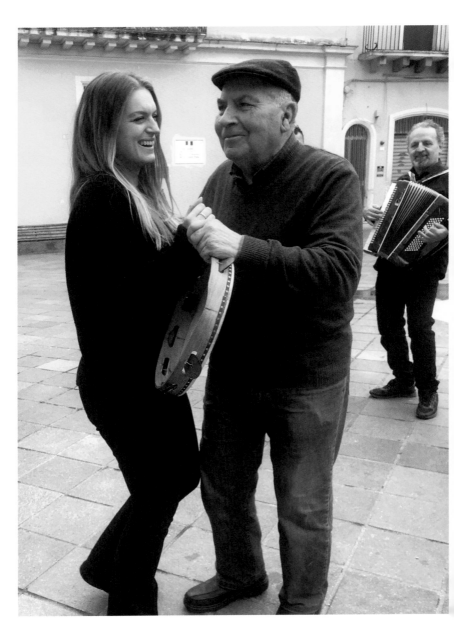

THE ORIGINS OF
pizzica

Part of the larger *tarantella* family, *pizzica* is the music originally played to accompany the therapeutic rite known as tarantism; traditionally, women who were thought to have been bitten by a tarantula were cured by dancing until the poison was expelled from their bodies. *Pizzica* today, however, is simply a popular dance, usually involving two people, accompanied by tambourines, harmonicas and accordions. The singing is always in dialect, and so has managed to remain very specific to local areas in Puglia.

If you manage to travel to Puglia during the month of August, try to get your hands on a calendar for the '*Festa della Taranta*', a popular music festival focused on *pizzica* and *taranta*. It lasts about a month, and each day it takes place in a different town. It's a great opportunity to learn about popular folk music, try food from the area and get involved with some of the dancing and singing with the locals. And if you really want to see how Italians live the philosophy of Dolce Far Niente to the fullest, this is the perfect occasion: summer heat, music, delicious food, rivers of wine, kids running and screaming all over the place and no sense of time whatsoever.

(FOOD) FESTIVALS
Sagre

In the past, *sagre* used to be more about religion than food, but Italians being Italians manage to transform any occasion into a food-related one. So while these festivals still have religious connotations (usually the fair is dedicated to the patron saint of the town it's in), they are usually all about giving exposure to a local food, often bearing the name of that specific food.

Traditionally, *sagre* were small fairs confined to the local inhabitants, but today they have become an important tourist attraction all over the country. And if you think about it, is there anything better than a small-town fair that brings family and friends together with music and great food? I don't think so.

Most of these fairs are held in the summer months, so people can be comfortable outdoors. However, some do take place in the colder months as well. A great way to find out about them is by going to the town centre and looking for the posters which are usually plastered all over the place. On the following page I have listed some of my favourite *sagre* in Italy.

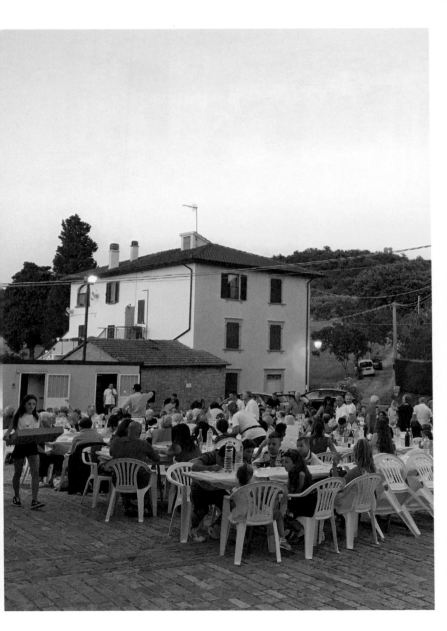

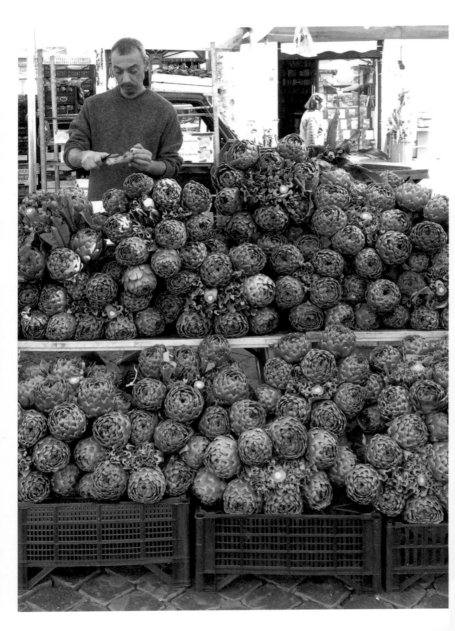

- **Sagra dell'uva (Grape Fair),
30 September–3 October in Marino, Lazio**
This is the only *sagra* I know of where actual wine pours out of the town's fountains. One of Italy's liveliest, the food that accompanies the wine at this fair is usually *porchetta* (roasted pork) sandwiches and *ciambelle al mosto* (sweet cookies made with raisins). Grapes and vines are placed all over the town as decoration.

- **Sagra del carciofo (Artichoke Fair),
10–12 April in Ladispoli, Lazio**
People in Rome (and all the towns that surround it) are obsessed with artichokes, but who would have thought there could be a whole fair dedicated to these tasty vegetables? Well, here you can try them in all kinds of dishes, while listening to local music and sipping on delicious wine.

- **Sagra del peperoncino (Hot Pepper Fair),
9–13 September in Diamante, Calabria**
This is the hottest fair in Italy (literally). This region of Italy is renowned for its delicious hot peppers and this is the perfect occasion to taste all of their traditional 'spicy' dishes.

- **Sagra della polpetta (Meatball Fair),
4–7 August in Grottaglie, Puglia**
Few things could beat a whole fair dedicated to meatballs! In this part of Italy, they are made with a mixture of different meats, parsley and cheese and then fried. This town is also known all over Italy for its beautiful ceramics, so the fair has amazing meatballs, beautiful plates, wine and traditional music.

MOVIES AND TV
Cinema e televisione

In Italy, the TV is constantly on. It serves as sort of a background noise for most homes, restaurants and bars, and people often feel weird switching it off. Back when TVs first appeared in Italian homes, it was a great way to learn about different countries, watch the news and listen to people speaking what was considered 'proper' Italian (as opposed to dialect – see p. 60). Sadly, today it's pretty much filled with garbage and reality shows.

The TV also plays an important role when it comes to mealtimes. Italians don't like sitting down to a meal on their own, but of course many people end up eating alone during the week because of different work schedules, so they use the TV for company. Many of the more 'traditional' restaurants in Italy will also have a TV on for their customers to watch while eating. Which reminds me of one of my favourite restaurants in the countryside region of Umbria: a small truck stop on the side of a main highway. (In Italy, truck drivers tend to eat the very best food available, so if you see a bunch of trucks parked outside a restaurant, run right in – they will probably serve some of the best food you have ever eaten in your life.) As soon as you walk inside, you will see a seemingly infinite number of men, all sitting alone at tiny tables facing the entrance. You might think they are staring at you, but what they are really doing is watching the large TV that is perched right above the entrance. Thankfully, Italy also has some of the most beautiful and rich cinematic history in the world. And Italians still love a good 'movie night' a few times a week. People in Italy still have a very strong attachment to older movies, especially those from the 50s and 60s. After the war, people wanted to get their minds off the bad things in life and used movies as a diversion.

I feel one of the best ways to get to know a country and its culture is through their movies, so I've compiled a list of some of my favourites. Most of these are available for purchase online, and some are even on YouTube.

Ladri di biciclette, **directed by Vittorio De Sica, 1946** This is a perfect view of the lives of Italians right after the Second World War. It's the story of a father and son, Antonio and Bruno, running desperately through Rome trying to find the father's stolen bicycle. One of my favourite scenes is when father and son sit down at a trattoria and order a *mozzarella in carrozza* (fried bread slices with mozzarella filling) – a symbol of hope for a new life after the war.

Domenica d'agosto, **directed by Luciano Emmer, 1950** The movie is simply a day at the beach for a Roman family, but the beauty of their packed lunch makes it exceptional. An explosion of spaghetti, wine, *frittata*, *porchetta* and prosciutto shows us the cheerful side of post-war Italy.

Roma, **directed by Federico Fellini, 1972** The story of a provincial man (who is actually Fellini himself) and his relationship with the eternal city. The movie is known for its outdoor dining scene in a piazza, filled with crowded tables, kids screaming and endless dishes of typical Roman food.

Non ci resta che piangere, **directed by Roberto Benigni and Massimo Troisi, 1984** This is one of the few movies that actually makes me laugh out loud. Two men are transported back from the twentieth century to 1492, and while at first they can't believe what is happening, they take it as an opportunity to speak to Leonardo da Vinci, stop Columbus on his journey and, of course, fall in love. The movie is more like a series of sketches, so it's really easy to follow and is great if you want to start learning some Italian.

Il Postino, **directed by Michael Radford and Massimo Troisi, 1994** This is my earliest movie memory. I remember watching it with my dad in our living room in Rome. The story revolves around Mario, a postman from a small fishing village on an island off Sicily. Most of the island's population is illiterate, so the only person getting mail is Pablo Neruda (the writer and poet), in exile with his wife. A beautiful friendship is born between Mario and Pablo that transcends the social classes. Gorgeous scenery, amazing music, poetry and an ending that makes it even more incredible.

CARD GAMES

Giocare a carte

If you've ever seen a group of people playing cards in Italy, you might have noticed that the cards themselves don't look like your standard ones with hearts, spades, clubs and diamonds. Italian cards have all sorts of names: *Trentine, Trevisane, Bresciane* and, the most popular of all (and my personal favourite), *Napoletane*. A deck comprises a total of forty cards divided in four suits: *coppe* (cups), *denari* (golds), *bastoni* (clubs) and *spade* (swords).

Card-playing is very popular in Italy. People of all ages play, both men and women, and, to me, it is the epitome of Dolce Far Niente. While it's more common to see men playing in public, women often play in the privacy of their homes or a club. In smaller towns, every single coffee bar will have a group of men sitting either outside or inside playing for a few hours each morning and afternoon. They only play for points, never for money. However, things do often get heated. Whenever I am feeling stressed or overwhelmed, I like to go to my local coffee bar and watch the men playing for a while; it's oddly relaxing and definitely very entertaining.

The most popular games are *Scopa, Briscola* and *Tresette*. *Scopa* (meaning 'broom') is the easiest one to play, as well as the most common, and taking a *scopa* during the game literally means 'sweeping' all the cards off the table. The game can be played by two or four people, and the cards can be found online and in any tobacco shop or newspaper stand in Italy. Get yourself a deck and become a master *scopa* player; it will be much more fun to see the men in small Italians towns play if you understand the game, and you will look like a pro if they ask you to join them!

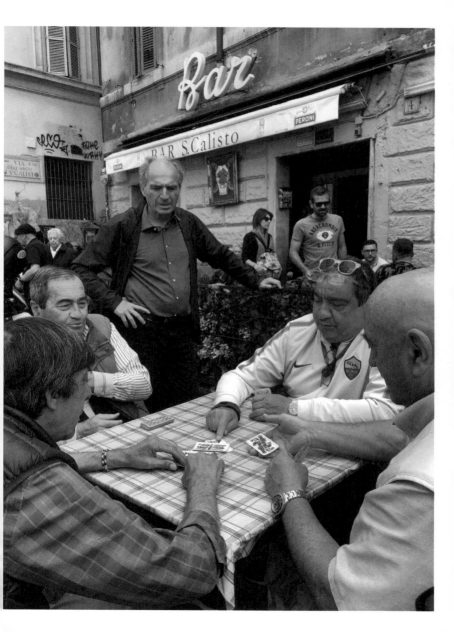

ICE CREAM

Gelato

I DECIDED TO INCLUDE THIS HERE, RATHER THAN IN THE PREVIOUS CHAPTER, BECAUSE EATING *GELATO* IS LESS ABOUT FOOD AND MORE ABOUT RELAXING AND JUST ENJOYING THE MOMENT.

Some of my earliest food memories are associated with *gelato*. When I was a baby, my mom took me to her preferred *gelateria* in Rome – the place where she had her first bite of *gelato* on her very first trip to the eternal city. I can clearly remember my little cup filled with artisanal wild strawberries and rice (yes, they have an amazing rice flavour, similar to rice pudding). Needless to say, this is still my favourite place in Rome and I have never changed my flavour choice.

When I grew a little older, I also became obsessed with *gelati confezionati*, a variety of pre-packaged (and probably filled with preservatives) ice creams available at every bar in Italy. They are kept in old-fashioned rectangular fridges, and I would spend hours just staring at them, trying to figure out which one I wanted. Every kid has their own favourite, but the excitement of feeling like an adult and getting to pick my own never got old.

As with everything food-related in Italy, there are rules for eating your *gelato*:

1. **Time of day** *Gelato* is never to be eaten in the morning, but is always appropriate after lunch or dinner as dessert or in the afternoon as a snack. It usually accompanies the afternoon *passeggiata* (see p. 131).

2. **_Cono o coppetta_** As soon as you enter a *gelateria* you will be asked if you want a cone (*cono*) or cup (*coppetta*). Once you have decided this, you can choose the size. Most Italians prefer the smallest.

3. **Flavours** There is no such thing as scoops in Italy. No matter the size of cup or cone you choose, you are always allowed three flavours: and yo   will be served a little of each with a flat spoon. You are expected to order at least two flavours; if you only order one, the person behind the counter will look really confused as to why you are depriving yourself of two other flavour choices.

4. **Samples** There is no such thing as *gelato* sampling when in Italy. It can feel risky, but you are expected to just go in, have a quick look at the flavours and pick the three that attract you the most. You could end up with one flavour you don't love, but hey, there are worse things in life!

5. **_Panna?_** The person behind the counter will always ask if you would like some *panna* (whipped cream) on your *gelato*. If you are sure you're in a good place (and by 'good place' I mean somewhere where the gelato is homemade), always say yes, it's usually delicious, and never the terrible stuff that comes out of a can!

While Italians generally prefer to sit down in order to truly enjoy their food, *gelato* is the one thing you are allowed to eat while slowly strolling around (and the key word here is *slowly*) because if it's not eaten right then and there, it will melt in your hands.

THE GARDEN
Il giardino

Most people in Italy live in small homes or apartments, so they don't usually have a big garden to take care of. Italians love to have as much greenery around them as possible though, even if it's clear there is no space for it, and if you take a walk around Rome, you will notice tiny terraces filled to the brim with flowerpots and herbs, vines climbing across buildings and random fig trees on every corner. Italians like most things in life to be beautiful and that extends to something as simple as a terrace in the big city. The most popular plant on terraces is geraniums: you will see them in all colours imaginable, even popping out of windows when there is no terrace available.

Back in 1990, my dad decided to plant a small fig tree on the corner of our building in Rome, to see if it would make it in the midst of all the cobblestones and traffic. Twenty-nine years on, it is as tall as a three-storey building and is laden with figs in the summer, making it a neighbourhood attraction. We all love the fig tree very much and take care of it as best we can, which might mean pruning it every now and then. When a new (and not-so-nice) neighbour moved in down the road a few years ago he decided to call the police after 'catching' my dad pruning the tree. (While it's illegal to plant anything on Rome's public streets, it's also illegal to take anything down; yes, Rome has rules that make absolutely no sense.) When the police arrived and listened to my dad's side of the story, they laughed and told the neighbour to leave both my dad and the fig tree alone.

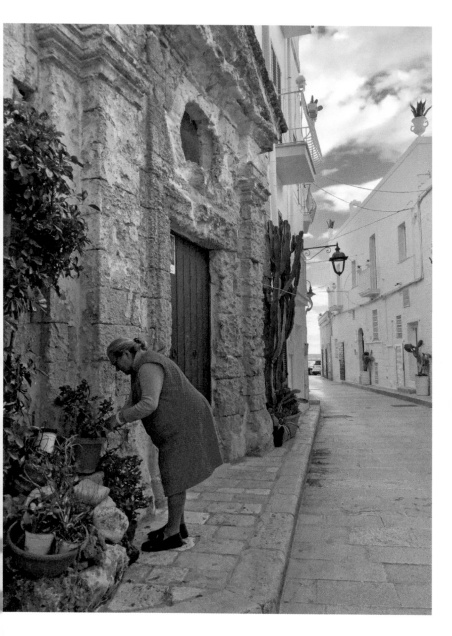

SPORTS
Attività fisica

Italians are not known to be the 'sportiest' of people, yet they all follow football, or soccer, as if it were a religion.

As soon as a child is born in Italy, they immediately become an avid follower of their family's preferred football team and will, in turn, pass on that love and adoration to their own children later in life. While this passion can be quite extreme, at the end of the day, it's all about a feeling of community and belonging to a social network – because as obsessed as they all are with their teams, they also all love each other, regardless of which teams they support. This is also why most people prefer to watch the games outside of the home, at a restaurant, bar or club: watching and then discussing a game with strangers or friends is considered a social activity, just as much as drinking a coffee together or sharing a meal.

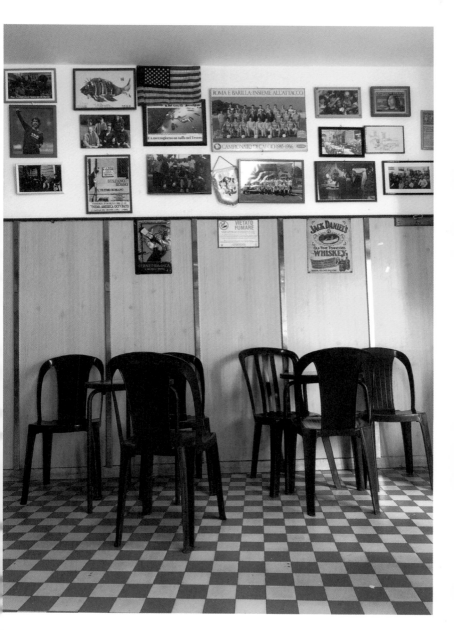

HOW CAN I INCORPORATE SOME OF THESE CONCEPTS INTO MY LIFE?

1

Have an aperitivo

Try making a point of meeting up with a colleague or friend after work a couple of times a week for an *aperitivo*. In Italy, this is not so much about the food and drink, but a way for people to connect with each other while 'disconnecting' their brains after a long day at work. If you can't find a bar you like near your workplace or home, try hosting it at your place. It can be a quick nibble and drink or it can easily become a casual dinner by adding a few simple dishes.

2

Learn an Italian card game (or something similar)

Nothing says Dolce Far Niente like a group of people playing card games for hours and hours. In Italy, people completely lose track of time doing this, sitting outside a coffee bar. Card games are entertaining, but also benefit our emotional and mental health, keeping our minds active and boosting concentration, while providing a social outlet too – all of which are fundamental to a happy and healthy life. But if cards aren't your thing, choose another activity that will keep you entertained without switching on the TV or your phone. Pick up a newspaper and make an effort to read it from front to back or try completing a couple of crossword puzzles.

3

Take a break

Life can often feel overwhelming, but nowadays we tend to think that it's better to just push through and ignore that feeling of being swamped rather than acknowledge the fact that we may need a break from whatever it is that is stressing us out. Whether it's at work

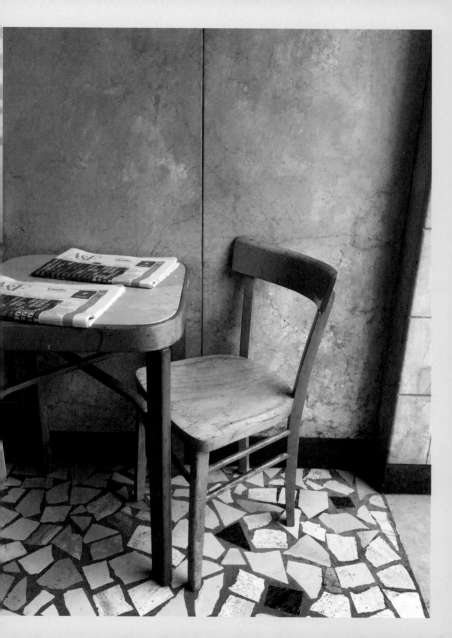

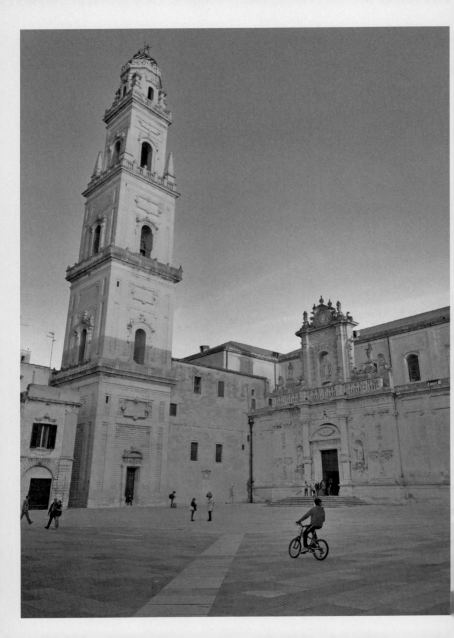

or at home, take time for yourself when your body and mind are telling you that it's needed. A quick walk, a longer lunch break or a short coffee break will reboot your sense of wellbeing.

4

Bella figura

Italians like to look good whenever they leave the house, even if it's just to buy some milk down the road. They truly believe that life is better when you look better, simply because you will feel better. When it comes to dressing the Italian way, choose quality over quantity: invest in a few key pieces that will last you a long time and will work for any occasion. Shoes are also very important: you will never see an Italian leave the house in flip-flops (except for the beach).

5

Seek out *sagre*

You might not be near enough to Italy to go to *sagre* there, but you can visit local festivals. These days food festivals abound, and it's a great way to connect with your local community. Or get together with your neighbours to plan your own community fair. Pick your favourite food as a theme, add some good music and make it a yearly event by recreating a mini-*sagra* in your own home, inviting all your friends over to eat (and drink) the night away.

6

Enjoy some beach time

There is something to be said for being outside near a body of water. It's not for nothing that Italian doctors recommend this to their patients at least once a year. They may cite the therapeutic benefits of breathing in the iodine from the sea water, but just letting your eyes rest on the distant horizon is a tonic in itself. If you can make it to the sea, fantastic. If not, then shoot for a river or lake. Try to include friends and family, and be sure to take a packed lunch with you.

AND FINALLY ...

Per Finire ...

I hope by now that I've been able to convey that Dolce Far Niente is not about 'doing nothing'; rather, it's about letting go of anxiety and the pressure to be constantly productive, and learning to be a little more 'bored'. In this case, boredom is not a negative thing – it's part of a broader picture of maintaining creativity and pushing aside the overwhelming in order to make space for 'real' thoughts.

While writing this book, I've actually learned a lot myself, so to conclude, here are a few final takeaways – things that I hadn't, perhaps, previously fully understood and that I think can be useful to anyone wanting to bring positive change to their lives.

Find pleasure in the ordinary.
In order to live life to the fullest, I truly believe it's important to make every day an 'extraordinary' one by finding joy in the smaller things – a coffee at the same place every morning, eating gnocchi every Thursday or enjoying the warm sunlight on a bench for ten minutes a day.

Work hard, but remember to prioritise.
To work well, you need to feel well. And this means maintaining a certain level of self-care, whether that's taking a longer weekend, reading a book in the park, going for a walk on the beach or by a river or enjoying an *aperitivo* or glass of wine after work.

Ditch the guilt.
Feelings of guilt are often strongest when we're doing something for ourselves – when we sit down to have a coffee instead of cleaning up the house or eat our lunch at the park instead of answering emails at our desks.

Italians have an innate skill for 'letting go' and doing whatever it is they would rather do, and this is something we can all learn from. It's not about being lazy; it's about simply allowing yourself to find the perfect balance between work and play in order to live a life full of meaning.

Use routine to your advantage.
For Italians, having a routine is beneficial to both physical and mental health: it takes away the stress of worrying about when or how you're going to get things done because you manage your time effectively; it improves your sleep (whether a daily nap or how you sleep at night), and, of course, your diet – because you factor in grocery shopping and cooking time (in Italy there is no such thing as 'I don't have time to cook'). So find a routine that works for *you* and stick to it.

Spend lots of time with family and friends.
Italians have a very strong connection with friends and family, often mixing the two together. No matter where you are from or how old you are, it's important to establish a network of friends and stay in touch with your family. Italians tend to have the same group of friends from a very young age, but as you go through life, things change, and so friends often change too. Pick up a new hobby and get to know like-minded people who enjoy doing the same activities. Call some of your closest friends and meet up for an after-work drink, making it a weekly routine.

Be open and welcoming.
One thing that still surprises me about Italians is their ability to make you feel welcome and loved as if you are their own blood. People I've known for just a few hours have invited me into their homes to sit at their dinner tables, with their family, making me feel indescribably loved. This is one of the positive aspects of lacking a sense of personal space – they share everything,

from their food to their emotions and their homes. Try being a little more generous in your day-to-day life – I assure you, it will all come back to you one day.

Live and love.
Italians put love into everything they do, whether it is singing their way to work in the mornings, making a pot of coffee for a loved one or picking the perfect head of lettuce at the market. A life filled with schedules and stress can become 'lighter' by appreciating the beauty and love that surround you.

Use food to bring you happiness.
As you've seen, food in Italy is about much more than simple sustenance. While the benefits of a Mediterranean diet are well recognised, the traditions and routines that surround it are just as important. We all experience times of extreme stress, but Italians manage to set all that aside when they sit down at a table to eat. Try making at least one meal a day a sacred and happy affair, focusing fully on the food that's in front of you and the company you are with.

Slow down.
Perhaps the most important thing I've learned is the importance of slowing down. This means: single-tasking rather than continuously switching between a multitude of tasks; making space in between appointments or activities, so you won't feel you are constantly on the go; living in the moment and being more mindful of whatever it is you are doing in that moment; focusing on the people around you, so your mind doesn't wander to things you need to do or what you want to say next; eating more slowly so that your food will taste better and you will feel fuller on less food. If you can manage to slow down – doing as the Italians do by putting less emphasis on the concept of time – you will really connect with the people in front of you,

instead of just meeting them, and, in the long run, you will find love, beauty and pleasure in all you do.

Growing up in Italy was amazing for so many different reasons. Some are more obvious, like the delicious food, shining sun and beautiful architecture. But others, the less obvious ones – those I've described throughout the book and have always taken for granted – are the ones I am truly thankful for. Dolce Far Niente is a lifestyle, and it underpins each and every single aspect of the Italian way of living, from the moment we leave our homes and make our way to school as kids, to meeting our friends for a drink after work when we are grown up.

If there is one simple way to put it, Dolce Far Niente is about taking things slow, even if it feels like we live in a world where everything seems to move so fast. We have too much, yet we often think we are missing something, making us feel empty and unsatisfied. From my life in Italy, I've come to realise that it's the small things in life that bring happiness: family, friends, a walk on the beach and a plate of home-cooked pasta.

Dolce Far Niente is about living in the present – savouring every moment as if it's the last – while remembering that life is an infinitely precious gift. Because life truly is beautiful. Let's never forget that.

ACKNOWLEDGMENTS

This book was made possible thanks to so many people. First of all, my amazing parents who allowed me to grow up in Italy, the country that surrounds me with constant beauty and delicious food. I want to thank Italy, my country and my first love – thanks to you, I've mastered the art of Dolce Far Niente and learned how to appreciate the beautiful things in life. I also want to thank all my friends who have stuck by me in good and bad times: you are the ones I love 'doing nothing' with. Finally, thank you to all the 'older' strangers I have met over the years – you have allowed me to dream about how life used to be through your stories, and reminded me what the important things in life truly are.

Thanks to all the lovely people over at HarperCollins, especially Carolyn Thorne, Georgina Atsiaris and James Empringham.

ABOUT THE AUTHOR

Sophie Minchilli is a half-Italian half-American 'Italy lover', born and raised on pasta in the cobblestoned alleys of Rome. She currently runs food tours all over Italy, mainly focusing on Rome, Puglia and Umbria. She likes to show her clients the 'real Italy', often leading them behind the scenes and into the homes of locals. She graduated in London with a degree in Communications at LCC.